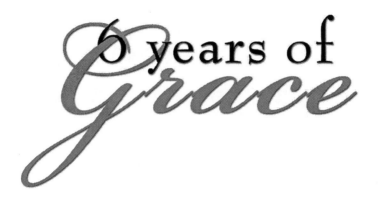

6 years of Grace

Jennifer Sokol

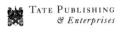

TATE PUBLISHING
& Enterprises

Dedication

For my mother
whose love will sustain me for all eternity

Acknowledgments

Thank you to all those who nudged me forward and encouraged me to share these episodes. To Jackie O'Ryan, my dear friend and first reader, who helped me envision possibilities beyond my imagination. To Louise Marley, who generously offered her time and wisdom, and who continues to inspire me by her gifts. To all those who prayed, silently enabling the flow of grace. And finally, to my father who was there for me at every moment, supporting, editing, humoring. Thank you, Dad, for your unwavering love.

Contents

Foreward

One of life's most difficult tests is to be there for someone in need, day in and day out. After ten years in a cloistered Carmelite monastery, Jenny Sokol left the religious life and was available when her mother had a serious life-changing stroke.

There was no confusion in Jenny's mind. She heard the call plainly and responded without doubt. Her father, Vilem Sokol, former University of Washington Professor and Director of the Seattle Youth Symphony, was unable to provide the kind of constant care his wife needed. All of her nine siblings were now grown and gone, leading lives of their own.

A once vibrant and dynamic woman, Agatha could no longer command her own body. But her life was far from spent and Jenny was determined to help her live the rest. Over six years, Jenny was her mother's caregiver, selflessly performing the necessary messy chores, sometimes in a state of exhaustion, sometimes in a flurry of playful chaos, almost always with her characteristic faith-filled tenderness.

There are over 25 million family caregivers in America today. Daily they launder, clean, groom, transfer, hold and sustain. This book documents one faith-filled journey through the labyrinth of caring. We watch as gifts are exchanged between the giver and receiver and see the lines that define the two grow blurry.

God lures into the desert hearts that are willing to be made tender. This daughter's willingness was remarkable and her desert tenderness bloomed beyond imagining.

When Jenny reclaimed her heart after her journey, she gave it back again to the world. This small book proves that when we give, even though our hearts may be heavy, they become channels for a love far greater than our own.

Jackie O'Ryan
Writer, Editor and Social Advocate

The First Day

~⟨⟨⟩⟩~

"Just hold her really close to you."

The therapist's words rang loudly in my head as I struggled to transfer my mother Agatha from the front seat of the station wagon to the wheelchair in the driveway at home. Having already dropped her in the hospital room that morning, I was terrified, and wondered, *Can I do this?* I kept imaging the way Molly, Mom's favorite therapist, had demonstrated the technique so confidently back in the hospital parking lot. Molly's final words to me were a light, "Just hold her really close . . ."

Poor Mom, 72-years-old and crippled after a major left-sided stroke, retained no boosting power to stand. Her left arm and leg were useless. She needed me to be strong for her. Taking firm hold of the cotton transfer belt buckled around her full waist, I tried again, this time successfully lifting her to her feet. But my heart pounded. I hardly knew my right side from my left as I clung to her in a bear hug, blindly positioning her left knee between both of mine.

"Just a second, Mom, I've almost got it now. Ready?"

"Ready." On cue, she lifted her right foot, which clumped to the ground again.

I pulled her closer. "You need to step again. Can you?"

"Yes, fine."

With the next step, we continued our counter-clockwise rotation, focused on Mom's lifeless leg. *Don't drop her!* A final step, and she stood directly in front of the wheelchair. Reaching behind to grab the arm rest, she slowly bent forward and I eased her down onto the seat. Woosh! The thick pad cushioned the landing.

"Done," I sighed.

Meanwhile, Dad, waiting silently nearby, handed me the wheelchair's left footrest and observed as I hooked it into place. Snap! It was secure, but not me. With endless details to manage, my interior plea was constant. *Mother of God, help me.*

Now, like this. Reaching under Mom's left knee with one hand, I grasped the lip of her ankle-top athletic shoe with the other. Substitutes for regular shoes, these white clompers supported her weak ankles after the stroke. I carefully lifted her disabled foot onto the footrest and released the wheelchair brakes. With Dad at my right, I stepped behind Mom and guided her to the front door. She was finally home with us again, October 30, 1992.

But no sooner had we bumped over the threshold, than I was seized with more panic. *Mom needs 24-hour care!* The door clicked shut behind us. Somehow, bringing her home had finally brought that glaring fact home as well. The awful truth was that Dad and I were unprepared.

I stood beside the coat closet in the front hallway and reached down, slipping Mom's left arm from the coat sleeve. "Here," I instructed, nudging her upper body forward.

Leaning, she attempted to boost herself as I yanked the slick, salmon-colored fabric from beneath her. Sitting back, she squirmed free of the right sleeve, then froze, unable to continue.

She can't do anything! Overwhelmed, questions flooded my mind. *What will I do, working at a downtown print shop? How can Dad do full-time nursing? He doesn't even know how to do transfers. What if I leave Mom with him tomorrow? Can he manage for six hours alone? What if I stay? Am I competent to care for her?* I didn't know. Sheer necessity demanded that I return to the present moment.

I turned and handed the raincoat to Dad. "Could you take this, please? Mom needs to lie down."

Taking it, he headed out the door to retrieve the rest of her things in the car.

But Mom was not thinking of rest. "Take me to the phone, Jenny." Her voice quavered with urgency. "I need to call the doctor."

"Why?"

"To find out about nursing agencies. I need someone to take care of me."

My heart sank. "I didn't realize how much care you would need until we got home, Mom."

"I know. But I really need someone. Please, wheel me to the kitchen."

By now it was late on a Friday afternoon, so the call had to be made before the doctor's office closed. I pushed the wheelchair down the long terrazzo hallway and parked Mom near one of the tall picture windows in the kitchen. Bewildered, I handed her the cordless phone, watching as she one-handedly punched out the number in her weakened condition. She lifted the phone to her right ear, hidden behind a white, cotton headband, and pressed it to her straight, shoulder-length silver hair. Her conversation with the nurse began. "Hello, Helen?"

Half listening, my gaze wandered out the window. The familiar view of hills, blanketed with evergreens, were drenched beneath a gloomy sky of rainy Seattle weather. Like a storm, Mom's stroke had triggered a labyrinth of confusing questions and unresolved emotions within me. As if mirroring my inner cloudiness, the day's misty conditions hung as a perfect reflection. I remembered the day I had left a Carmelite monastery the year before, and returned home—the tears, confusion, and loss. After ten years in a cloister, adjusting to lay life had been difficult enough. Now what was happening? What was God asking of me?

Mom's conversation ended. Looking up, she sadly announced, "They can't get anyone. Everything is closed for the weekend."

"Closed?" Sinking within, the word hollowed out hopelessness, and I stepped to Mom's side. "Now what do we do?"

She handed me the phone and closed her eyes. Wearily, she laid her head in her right palm, her elbow balanced on the wheelchair's black arm rest. Knowing she had begun to pray, I followed suit, listening within.

A dinner conversation at once flashed into my mind, one shared with my parents several weeks previously. That evening, Mom was speaking of a friend who had just been admitted to a nursing home. Since I had recently spoken with a few of my sisters regarding our parents' future care, I felt compelled to bring it up with Mom and Dad, explaining, "I want you to know that if anything happens to you, we won't put you in a nursing home. We'll take care of you."

Startled, Mom looked up and set her fork down. "You don't have to do that!"

"But we want to," I said. "It won't be a problem."

Strangely, as I spoke, I knew I would play a key role in the process of care, but I didn't understand how. Continuing no further, as quickly as the conversation began, it ended, though having touched a deep place in all of us.

I didn't think about it again until two weeks later when I returned home from work and discovered Dad's fateful note taped up on the wall just inside the back door: "Mom fell in the bathroom this morning. The doctor thinks she had a stroke. We're at the hospital."

I gasped, suddenly recalling the dinner conversation as if a prophecy had been fulfilled. I stared at the note, wondering, *Am I Mom's caregiver?* But I didn't hear the answer, or want to—I was too traumatized.

Trauma continued as I entered the ICU room at the hospital that evening and found Mom flat down in bed, her face flushed with fever, and her brow furrowed with pain. Years of high blood pressure, a heavy body weight, and emotional strain had taken their unfortunate toll. Dad nodded for me to speak.

"Hi, Mom."

Her eyelids flickered.

Moving nearer, I slipped my fingers into her sweaty palm. "I'm so sorry this happened. How are you feeling?"

"My head is throbbing," she responded weakly. "I feel like I'm burning up, and I'm completely nauseous." Her voice, lower in pitch, had a frightening, gravely tone.

"Is there anything I can do?"

"Maybe you could help me to sit up." Her eyes half opened. "My back is so sore."

Dad and I moved into action. While he reached, lifting her upper body from the mattress, I climbed up behind her and crouched on my knees at the head of the bed. Mom's feverish body lay like smoldering embers against my own.

In the next minute, she said, "Thank you. Now I think I'd better get back down." She never complained.

The rest of her five-week hospital stay offered little light to dispel my darkness. Strokes and their effects were almost entirely unknown to me. I struggled to comprehend new terms and medical explanations. I watched Mom labor daily through physical therapy. At the end of each session, she was exhausted, curled up on her side on a blue exercise mat. When the thought recurred about being her caregiver, I wondered, *Should I? Can I?* But the more enigmatic question loomed stronger: *Will she walk again?* Everything depended on that.

We questioned therapists about it many times. Their replies were invariably vague. "Maybe." Or, "It's hard to tell."

When Dad inquired about the possibility of caring for Mom at home, his only response came from a nurse who stood by Mom one afternoon, changing the bed linens.

"You have a nice bed, don't you?" she asked, mechanically lifting the sheet away.

"Yes," Dad replied.

"Well, that will probably be fine." She tossed the dirty linen into a white canvas bag and glanced up. "Otherwise, Agatha will have to go to a nursing home."

But Mom would hear nothing of it. After the nurse had left, she pleaded, "Please, no nursing home. I just couldn't bear it."

Dad and I decided to do our best and care for her at home. It seemed a reasonable possibility and no one objected.

Then, as Mom and I continued our silent vigil in the kitchen, I felt a sense of hope, and at the same moment, another presence nearby—a spiritual one. Immediately, I recognized it to be Mary, God's Mother, gently but firmly encouraging me: *You're the nurse.* Strengthened, I felt new confidence, realizing I would be a good nurse for Mom; we would work well together.

My job came to mind. *What about that? Should I keep it?*

The only answer seemed to be to let it go, at least for now.

And the rest of my life? How long will Mom need me?

For all I knew, her condition might linger for years. But that, it seemed, was not mine to know. At the moment I was simply being asked to step out in faith and give my everything for my mother, just like Mary who gave her everything for God. Convinced by what I understood was a call, I was ready to answer; Mom was waiting.

Looking down, I quietly said, "I'll do it, Mom. I'll be your nurse."

Astonished, she looked up, meeting my eyes. "Oh, I don't want to ruin your life!"

"You won't ruin my life." For the first time in weeks, I felt joy as I leaned over, caressing her head to my shoulder. "I want to do this. I'll take care of you."

Just then, Dad joined us.

Renewed, Mom looked up and excitedly informed him, "Jenny said she'd take care of me, Bill."

Surprised, he wondered about my job. "Don't you think you should keep it?"

"No. Mom is my job now."

Reaching, he wrapped me in a hug. Held within his tall, strong stature, I felt supported by what had always been the safest place in the world to me, Dad's arms.

Our commitment to one another was sealed. None of us carried illusions about the gravity of Mom's illness or unknown issues regarding her care. But we all knew that God would lead the way, guided by the loving hand of Mary. We only needed to take the next step.

That meant returning to the daunting task of settling Mom in, and she was tired. Stepping behind the wheelchair, I guided her to the opposite end of the hallway where Dad and I scoped out the furniture arrangement in their bedroom.

"The bed table," I said, gesturing with my head toward the brown mahogany piece just inside the doorway. "It needs to go."

Lifting it away, Dad stepped aside and I eased the wheelchair into place. Backed against the wall, there was just enough room to transfer Mom into bed.

Shoes off, brakes on, transfer belt tightened. I reviewed my list and carried out each action. Pulling the bed covers back, I ignored my pounding heart and gripped Mom's transfer belt, lifting her to her feet. *Here we go again. Don't drop her!*

I swayed, moving in sync with her body, but she slumped, breaking the flow. I pulled her tighter, fighting to keep both of us upright. *And this will go on all day, everyday? Please, help us, Blessed Mother.*

Ready to sit, Mom reached behind and felt for the mattress. I let her down and swiveled her to a lying position, then sighed. The king-size bed, unable to raise or lower, was like a rock in comparison with the soft hospital bed she was used to. Pinned under the heavy quilt, she was miserable, even while claiming, "I can make do, Jenny." She wormed, attempting to shove the quilt from her chest and shift to a more comfortable position. She looked to her right, dubiously patting the middle of the bed. "I guess I can put things here—"

"No, Mom. Wait." Closing my eyes, I calculated her needs. *Without the use of her left arm, she needs a bed table on her functioning right side. She needs a lamp to switch on and off by herself. And privacy in a room by herself, everything set up for comfort.*

I looked at her again. "What about the bedroom next door? It might work better. At least you'll have a bed of your own, and we can arrange the furniture properly."

"That's fine, honey," she said matter-of-factly. "Now, I need the commode."

The commode! My first attempt, and already time for another transfer. I eyed the beige apparatus in the corner of the room, delivered by a rental company the day before. Pulling it alongside the bed, I frowned at the rust spots, which dotted the frame. I applied the brakes and rolled Mom up to the side of the bed.

She was embarrassed. "I'm sorry you have to do this, Jenny."

"Please, don't worry." Helping her with her pants, I kidded, reminding her of the thousands of times she had done the same for me as a baby. "You're just a little bigger now than I was then."

Settled back in the wheelchair, Mom waited while Dad and I rushed to prepare the small, unoccupied bedroom next door. We pulled the twin-size bed out from the corner of the room and tucked in lightweight blankets. I rolled in a wheeled tray to use as a bed table, covered it with a white bath towel, and set a small, brown-and-white lamp on top. Just as I plugged the cord into the wall, Dad wheeled Mom through the doorway. Bump! The wheelchair nicked the narrow frame.

"I'll take it from here." I stepped behind Mom. *Back the wheelchair against the wall, so the bed is on her right side.* I could hear Molly's voice again: "That way, Agatha can step with her right foot and move in the direction of the transfer." *Yes, this way . . . so far so good. Now, set the brakes . . . that's the next step, I think . . . or, was it . . . I'll never remember everything!* Mom leaned forward, grasping the right brake handle, and set it herself. I stepped in front of her and clamped down on the left.

"Here we go." I gripped the transfer belt and marked the countdown. "One, two, three."

On three, she staggered to her feet, pleading, "Watch that arm!" Quickly, she reached across her tummy and grabbed the free-swinging limb.

"Don't let go of me, Mom!"

While she sighed, I heaved, at last flouncing her to a prone position. She was safely down, but no better. The bed was horrible.

"I feel like I'm lying on a board."

"I know. You look like it." More desperate than

ever, I studied her frightened brown eyes. "You really need a hospital bed, Mom."

"Maybe you could call a rental place. But it will be hard to find anything open this late on a Friday."

She was right; our present plight was a tough one. A hospital bed would be needed for an extended period, and the cost for renting that long enormous. Pricey or not, Dad was soon on the phone and called several rental places. Returning, the news was bleak.

"I can't get anyone," he said. "Everything is closed for the weekend."

Closed? Again, the hopeless word sank with a thud.

But Mom was not discouraged. Digging into the pocket of her turquoise knit pants, she pulled out her black wooden rosary and laid it on her tummy. "Something will work out. I'll pray."

In the midst of the chaos, an occupational therapist arrived at the front door, carrying a shower bench. "Your Mom will need it," she said, hastily walking through the door and following me down the hallway. She scanned the two upstairs bathrooms and decided to use the shower in Dad's room for Mom. "Better for transfers."

She unhinged the glass door and suggested a plastic curtain replacement. Several suggestions followed about how to transfer Mom inside, including the use of a "slide board" as she called it, in my eyes, a perilous looking thing. "Just shuffle Agatha across," she explained, demonstrating the precarious procedure.

But between the skimpy looks of the narrow board and my lack of experience, I could only envision disaster. Either Mom or I would end up on the floor, and I was afraid that it wouldn't be me. I bargained. "What if I just use our current transfer method. Will that be all right?"

"Yes, fine," she replied. "Just take it slowly." Quickly, she lowered the slide board into her equipment bag and sealed the front flap. Turning, she waved as she headed toward the front door. "Gotta run now. Another appointment."

"Right . . ." I stared after her, dumbfounded by the abrupt departure. Glancing at the bench, my mind reeled. *Was there anything else I needed to ask? Can I safely do the transfer? I'm on my own . . . What next? Dinner.*

I ran into the kitchen and pulled open the refrigerator, lifting out cooking ingredients. *Chicken, carrots, potatoes.* In between frantic chopping, I made several 40-yard dashes down the hallway to check on Mom; her needs were constant.

"My legs can't move under these covers," she said, squirming as I adjusted the blankets. Two minutes later: "This pillow is too hard. Do we have something softer?" A minute later: "I need to get higher up on the bed. Could you and Bill please pull me up?"

"Okay." I reached under her shoulders to lift her, then gasped. "Oh no! I hear water boiling over on the stove."

I ran from the room.

At serving time, Dad wheeled Mom to her place at the kitchen table and clipped a white paper napkin under her chin. Lacking adequate hand control, like an infant, Mom needed a bib to catch food spills now. Dad secured the portable plastic tray onto the wheelchair and placed her plate of food on top. "There, sweetie."

But she eyed it warily and pointed to the table. "Could you put it there, instead?"

Dad and I looked at one another. Seated at her regular place at home, we both knew that Mom was feeling her lack of independence and fighting for even a small measure of dignity. She hated the tray. Granting her request, however, Dad removed it and watched the struggle.

Mom bobbed like a buoy, pressing forward with her upper body, straining to reach the fork. Repeatedly, the wheelchair banged the edge of the table. Finally, realizing the futility, she sat back, and sighed. "Okay, Bill, that's fine. I'll use the tray."

Bending, he replaced it and set her dinner plate back on top. We made the sign of the cross, offered grace, and began to eat our first meal together.

After dinner I carried a small package to Mom and set it on the table in front of her. "It came this afternoon," I explained, "from Aunt Shirley." The gift from her sister, I hoped, would boost her spirits. "May I open it?"

"Oh, I guess you have to," she said, quickly retracting her hand, instinctively extended to peel the packaging away.

Inside the box were four brightly colored, handmade flannel nighties designed in the style of hospital gowns.

"Oh, aren't they pretty!" Mom said, touching the first one with her fingertip as I held it up.

"Yes. And just in time. I've been wondering all afternoon what I would dress you in tonight. None of your regular nighties would have worked. Which one would you like to wear first?"

But she didn't answer. Looking past me, she pointed toward her room. "I need to get down. And I don't think I'll be able to get up again tonight. Hurry." She bowed her head, exhausted.

I glanced at the wall clock. *Only 7:30.* Lying flat on the miserable bed for hours, Mom's night was sure to be a grueling one. Any relief I could provide would be minimal. I stepped behind the wheelchair and waited for Dad, who pushed aside the small couch near the kitchen table. The wheelchair reduced every space.

Wheeling Mom toward her room, I mentally reviewed bedtime preparations. I visualized how the nurses had lifted her in the hospital, how they handled her limbs, undressed and bathed her. In the hospital, the process was complicated enough. But at home I was in charge, and felt the full weight of responsibility. I prayed through my fear, trusting grace and instinct to carry me through. *Hail Mary, full of grace . . .*

I angled the wheelchair through the doorway and parked Mom alongside the bed. Helping her up and down several times, I removed her clothing, then dampened a washcloth in the bathroom sink and carried it back, also balancing a toothbrush, a tube of toothpaste, and a paper cup filled with water. Mom scrubbed her face and brushed her teeth, struggling to reach the narrower, back corner of her mouth. She swished with water, then spit into a blue plastic hospital basin, which I held under her chin.

"Almost done," I said, setting everything down on the floor and kneeling at her feet. "I have to remove your socks."

But the thin cotton anklets clung stubbornly, and

my elbows burned as I leaned into the scratchy gold carpeting for support.

"You're doing fine, Little One," she said, calling me by my childhood nickname. I hadn't heard that in years.

"Maybe you'll be strong enough to transfer onto the commode and wash at the sink tomorrow night." The final sock slid from her toes and I sat up straight.

"Yes, that would be nice," Mom said, brightening at the thought.

But optimism faded as I stood and lifted her left arm to wash underneath it. She started, embarrassed by the smell. "That's horrible!"

"Your arm is always pressed against your side," I explained. "All we can do is wash it."

"It just hangs there, doesn't it?" Disturbed, she reached across her chest to examine the noticeable gap between her left shoulder socket and lower arm. The powerless muscles hung loosely and she fingered the hollow evidence, another offshoot of the stroke. "I don't know if it will ever be normal again."

Looking down, she massaged the soft lump, mysteriously formed on top of her left wrist. "The doctors don't know what it is. It's so odd. Do you think it's gone down any?"

"No, I don't think so." I picked up the pink-and-white nightie draped over the bedspread. Lifting Mom's left wrist, I slipped her arm through the short-sleeved opening. "The lump doesn't look that bad. Really."

I stepped behind her and fastened the nightgown together at the collar. *If only I could quell at least a portion of her anxiety.* Bending, I reached around and embraced her.

Pressing my cheek to hers, I said, "We're going to make it through this, Mom. I know we are."

Reassured, she reached up and placed her hand over mine. "Okay, I'm ready now. Let's do the transfer."

But the bed was no comfort as I let her down. She struggled to reach the bed table, craning to see over the top. "Where's my rosary? Could you hand it to me?" She reached behind her head and attempted to reposition the pillow. "It's hard to do with only one hand. Maybe you could find me a bigger pillow tomorrow."

Dad poked his head through the doorway. "Jenny, the phone is for you."

I glanced at Mom.

"Answer it," she said. "I'll be fine."

Calls had been coming in all afternoon, mostly from my nine siblings who were anxious to hear how things were going. Naturally, everyone was surprised to hear of my decision to be Mom's caregiver, especially since I had so recently left the monastery. After 10 difficult years in the religious life, involving a relentless journey of self-revelation, and the painful uncovering of sexual abuse in my early childhood, I returned home to seek healing and a new life. No one ever imagined caregiving in my future, much less me.

I listened to my sister now, who spoke over the phone.

"You know, you don't have to do this," she said. "This isn't your problem."

But I assured her, "It isn't a problem. I want to do it."

Concerned, she asked more questions, which led to more discussion. But like everyone else, she soon realized that my decision was a positive one, affecting not only Mom, but everyone in the family. We all knew that Mom was much happier at home, and would receive good care. I promised that.

"Just know that I'll be praying for you," my sister said.

"Thanks. I count on that."

I hung up the phone and returned to Mom who admitted being too exhausted to use the commode again. That worried me.

"After all, we have nurses orders, remember? You're supposed to use the commode once more before going to sleep."

"That was really awful in the hospital this morning, wasn't it?" she said, reminded of the incident when the "orders" were given.

Just before bringing her home, Mom and all of the family present were led into a large conference room to discuss her home care. But the only topics brought up by the hospital staff were Mom's incontinence and her chronic bladder infections. Seated at the head of the imposing table, Mom was silent, her head bowed in humiliation the whole time. Neither she nor anyone in the family wanted the matter discussed publicly. A private consultation with me would have sufficed. But with little control over the matter, we simply wrapped things up as quickly as possible after enduring an overly extended description of details.

Mom offered a solution for our present problem. "How about using a bedpan? But would you mind going out to buy it? We don't have one in the house."

I sighed. Faced with yet another challenge, I checked the clock. *Late. And the store will close soon. Can*

I make it on time? I looked at Mom, overwhelmed by her helplessness. "All right. But you'll have to put up with me again. I don't even know how to use a bedpan."

"That's all right. I'll teach you."

I ran down the hallway and grabbed my coat and purse, both lying on the floor near the back door. Calling out directions to Dad, I headed to my car, parked in the carport, and climbed in the front seat. For the first time that day I was alone, and shivered in the cold evening air.

Driving down the hill from our house, nighttime darkness only magnified how much in the dark I was feeling myself. Again, by God's mysterious design, everything in my life had changed, a difficult place to be. I drove under traffic lights, passed neon signs, and glanced up at brightly lit billboards. But my light was Mary, the faith-filled woman of Nazareth. Had not God changed everything in her life as well? Her story was much different than mine, but surely she had experienced a similar trial: facing uncertainty in the dark with God. Following her example, I offered my own difficulty, trusting that God would also lead me.

I turned into the store parking lot and looked up into the night sky. Suddenly, a quiet thought passed through my mind: *The Carmelites have a hospital bed.*

Yes, they do! I eased the car to a halt in a parking space and turned off the engine. *But I haven't thought about that bed since I helped to store it away. Is this our solution for Mom?*

Conveniently, the Carmelites lived nearby. The hospital bed had been donated to the community, but I never imagined using it for my own mother someday. Perhaps, I hoped, the nuns would loan it to us. I stepped from the car, filled with the luminous prospect, and completed my late night mission to the store.

The plastic shopping bag crackled in my hand, flapping against my leg as I flew through the back door at home. Picking up the phone, I dialed the monastery and spoke with the prioress, Sister Michael Marie, about the bed. "Do you think we could borrow it?"

"Absolutely," she replied, typically calm. "When would you like to pick it up?"

I practically shouted. "Thank you so much! How about tomorrow morning at ten?"

"Fine. We'll have it waiting."

Mom was exhausted, but relieved to hear the good news. She endured the first bedpan lesson, patiently instructing me, then watched as I carried a stack of laundry toward the door.

"Don't you think that could wait until tomorrow morning?" she asked.

"No, I'd better put in a load tonight." I headed down the hallway.

But only two steps down the stairs, she called me back, distressed. "Jenny, can you come?"

I bounded back to her side where she was looking up from her wet nightie, paper cup in hand. "I couldn't sit up to drink, so I spilled water all over me. Could you help?"

I changed her wet nightie, then called Dad in to help. As in the hospital, he lifted Mom while I scooted in behind her at the head of the bed. We were a curious trio, with me acting as a back rest, Mom sipping water, and Dad telling cheerful anecdotes.

"But we can't possibly keep this up," I said, stepping off the bed. "Tugging and lifting you this way all night, Mom? How about using that spill-proof cup in the kitchen. You know—the one you keep on hand for the grandchildren. Would you mind?"

"No, that's fine," she said. For the first time that day, she turned up a small smile. "It's called a Tommy Tippy."

I found "Tommy" in the cupboard above the kitchen sink. A faded turquoise bear decorated the white, two-handled surface, and three tiny drinking holes peppered the lip. Filling the toddler's cup with water at the sink, I pondered Mom and her total dependence upon God, upon me, and everyone. *She's like a child now . . . the greatest in God's kingdom.*

The clanking ice announced my approach as I carried the cup down the hallway. Handing it to Mom, she wrapped her fingers around the roomy handle and sipped easily, no spills. From then on, she always referred to her cup as "My Tippy."

Before leaving for the night, I went in search of a bell, something she could call me with. *Isn't that old brass one sitting on the shelf over the oven?*

Sure enough, there it was, way in the back, hidden among the clutter. I pushed aside a cardboard filing box, and sifted past a corroded garden hose nozzle, torn rubber gloves, a lettuce wringer, and a decorative stack of bread baskets. I grasped the bell's wobbly handle and rang it softly, also hearing Mom's voice from long ago.

During our growing years, she stood on the front porch of our home, vigorously tolling the same bell. "Children, time for dinner!" she called out in her high, operatic-like tone. We responded, clamoring down sidewalks and turned up the front walkway. Dashing up the porch stairs, we disappeared into the house, ready to devour our meal.

I carried the bell to her room now, and set it on the table. "Can you reach it?"

She grasped the handle. "Yes, this will work."

"Try to relax, then. You really need to sleep. Do you need anything before I go?"

"Maybe you could put a pony tail on top of my head." She fingered her hair. "I don't like all of this around my neck."

Her hair had been hidden beneath a wig for years, a way to conceal psoriasis. After the stroke the scaliness subsided, so she never wore a wig again. "Besides, it's too much of a bother," she told me in the hospital.

I gathered the fine strands into a rubber band and reminisced about her "wig days" during my teenage years. When visitors stopped by the house, catching her at a wigless moment, she escaped into the nearest room and closed the door behind her. Later, poking her head into the hallway to check if the coast was clear, she reemerged and put her wig back on.

"It's nice to see you with your real hair again," I said. "You're beautiful just the way you are."

"Really?" Self-consciously, she reached and adjusted the drooping left corner of her mouth. "Is it bad?"

"No." I removed her glasses and set them on the bed table. "I hardly notice, Mom. Now, promise to ring if you need me."

"I will." She wriggled, straining to reach the light switch at the base of the lamp, then snapped it off.

Dad retired to his room, and I headed for mine, located directly below Mom's. But with each step down the staircase, foreboding possibilities played through my mind. *What if I sleep through the bell? What if there's an emergency? What if Mom panics? What if . . . What if . . .*

I climbed into bed and stared at the ceiling. *Should I sleep upstairs?*

The answer came immediately, signaled by the bell.

I sprang from bed and back up the stairs. Rounding the sharp left corner at the top, I noticed Mom's light was already back on. I flew through her doorway. "What's wrong?"

"I can't reach the extra blanket," she sighed, looking toward me over her left shoulder. Her right palm rested on her forehead. "I'm worn out from trying."

"Well, this decides it." I adjusted her blanket and walked toward the closet. "I'm going to sleep in the living room."

"What! Then what will you use for a bed?"

"A sleeping bag, I guess." I opened the closet door and pulled down a navy blue one stored on the overhead shelf. Slipping it from the dusty cleaners bag, I unrolled it and draped it over my arm. "I just couldn't live with myself if I slept through your bell."

I poked through other closets in the house and located a couple of thin, foam rubber pads among the heaps. *These will do for a mattress . . . easy to roll up in the morning.*

I carried everything down the living room steps and stopped next to the piano. *Sleeping quarters.* With Mom just on the other side of the wall, her every move would be within hearing range. *Perfect.* I laid everything down and settled in—almost. The bell rang.

"Coming," I said, climbing from the sleeping bag.

But I was glad to be nearer. Later, zipped in for the final time that night, my prayers changed to gratitude as the sound of Mom's breathing relaxed down the hallway. The day's most welcome blessing, at last a few hours of peaceful sleep had come to visit my mommy.

The Second Day

Rising before sunrise, I pulled on my sweatpants and a sweatshirt, relishing the luxury of morning silence. I remembered it was Halloween, but instead of trick-or-treaters, visitors that day would be family and medical professionals. Like yesterday, I anticipated a hectic pace. I longed for a sense of confidence as I sat down on the living room rug to begin my stretching exercises, but inner tension dictated differently; I was afraid. Closing my eyes, I prayed for light. *Come, Holy Spirit. Help me to do the transfers. Will I ever learn?*

Practice was just in store as my reflections were interrupted—the bell rang.

I jumped to my feet and hastened toward Mom's room, noticing daylight filter through the hallway windows. The grotto just outside harbored a white statue of Mary, her hands folded in prayer, within a small wooden shrine. The living Mary, I knew, was with us.

"How do you feel?" I asked Mom, arriving at her side.

"My back is really sore." Squinting from pain, she attempted to thrust the covers aside. "Please, get me up."

"I have to wash you first," I reminded her, pulling back the blankets and draping them at the foot of the bed. "But I'll do it quickly."

Morning washings became routine after the stroke,

the result of Mom wearing disposable diapers. I carried the plastic wash basin into the bathroom and filled it with water. I picked up three fresh towels and carried everything back to Mom and rolled her over onto her right side.

The towel, I began, concentrating as I spread it underneath her. *Completely flat, no wrinkles. Now, the soap. . . this much.* I dribbled a small amount of the clear golden liquid into a dampened wash cloth, careful not to splash. Mom never spoke, conserving energy.

Finished, I rolled her up to a sitting position and smoothed the rumpled nightie over her knees. "Can you push off from the mattress?"

She nodded.

I reached around and buckled the transfer belt into place, warning, "This will be hard for both of us."

The bed was low and Mom bounced helplessly, pumping with her right hand to push off from the mattress. I gripped the transfer belt, pulling her toward me, but without success.

"C'mon, Mom, we can do it," I sighed, pausing to catch my breath. "Here we go, one more time. Ready?"

Leaning further back, I pulled harder, wincing at the sight of the transfer belt, which scraped up her exposed back. *This must be killing her!* With a final pull, I lifted her to her feet, then let her down onto the commode. Flop!

"Thank God that's over with," she said, wiping stray hairs from her eyes. I jounced her twice more to adjust her lopsided position. Then she rested.

I stepped to the closet and opened the door, scanning her greatly reduced wardrobe. *A few colorful pant outfits.* How different from her previous collection of pretty daytime dresses and elegant evening attire, all feminine and stylish. Fashion was solely about utility now. Therapists recommended only exercise type clothing. "You know, stretchy knit pants and sweatshirts," they said. "They're great for doing physical therapy, and you can grip the waistbands during transfers." Mom wore them every day.

I turned and faced her. "Which outfit would you like to wear?"

But she didn't reply. Deep in thought, she was looking down, stroking her left hand knuckles, as if disturbed.

"What is it? Is there something wrong?" I stepped closer and she looked up.

"I wish I could help."

"I know. I'd probably feel the same way if I were you."

Again, I noted the remarkable change in her facial countenance. After the stroke, the strain had disappeared and she was no longer the active woman I had always known, in control, doing for others, managing everything. Entirely vulnerable, she was helpless and needed compassion.

I squatted and took hold of her slender hands, brown-spotted with age. "It's okay, Tiny Person."

Her transparent gaze penetrated my soul. In approval of her new name, she squeezed my hand, sealing trust. Then she said, "I think I'd better stay in what I'm wearing. I'm too tired to get dressed. Why don't you just put the white sweater on me."

I lifted away the knit garment hanging on the back of the desk chair and slipped her hand through the left sleeve opening. I drew the sweater around her shoulders, waiting as she squiggled through the right sleeve herself. One-handedly she groomed her hair with a comb, letting me hold clumps of it while she worked through the snags.

Once transferred into the wheelchair, she stared down at her left knee, which jutted awkwardly into the right. "It angles badly, doesn't it?" She pushed the left knee outward, attempting to equalize the look.

I walked to the linen closet in the hallway and pulled out a thin pillow. Carrying it back, I folded it in half and propped it between Mom's thighs for support. The knees separated.

"They say the muscles will get stronger," she said, watching as I slipped on her footies. "Then the left leg will sit normally again, right?"

She reached down and released the brake handle. Grasping the wheelchair's stainless steel wheel rim, she tried to propel herself across the rug.

"The nappy texture is hard to push across," I said, seeing her fruitless effort. I stepped behind the wheelchair and pushed. "I'll take it from here."

In the hallway, she propelled herself, though slowly. She turned the wheel rim, stepping forward with her right foot, and inched toward the kitchen.

Dad stood from his place at the table when we arrived. "Would you like your breakfast now, sweetie?" He leaned down and kissed her.

While Dad settled Mom at her place, I walked to the kitchen counter and studied the array of medication bottles. *So many. Let's see . . . Cardizem, Coumadin, Potassium, Synthroid.* I picked up each bottle, reading and rereading the hospital discharge papers. Satisfied, I assigned the prescribed dosages in a little clump on the counter.

"You take these with breakfast," I told Mom, carrying a small fistful to her place. I set the pills beside the glass of apricot juice. "Then you take two more at noon, and another one at bedtime."

"Got it." Eager, she picked up the first pill.

"But don't forget to eat something first."

"Right." Quickly, she set the tablet back down.

Dad slipped the cereal bowl in front of her.

With two hands free, I scurried back to her room to tidy up. In the next minute, the back door closed, announcing a visitor.

"Hi, everyone!"

It was Anne, my oldest sister, as usual right on time to help.

I pulled the last wet sheet from Mom's bed and added it to the collection on the floor. Arms loaded, I carried everything down the hall.

"Hi, Anne," Mom said sweetly, smiling as she looked up from her cereal.

As the two embraced, so began the long succession of first-time home visits from each of the children. Life, we understood, would never be the same for Mom. But none of us would ever get used to seeing her as an invalid.

Anne turned and wiped her tears as she moved farther away from the table. "We're going to fix up your room, Mom," she said, masking her emotions. Then privately to me, "I don't want to upset her."

"That's very nice," Mom said, unaware of our

exchange. She looked down at her cereal bowl and shakily lifted the spoon. The milk trickled from the banana slice, running down her napkin. She followed its pathway with her eyes, ignoring our company. Recognizing her withdrawn, protected manner, I knew she had taken in her fill of emotional impact. For now, it was best to leave her alone.

At work in Mom's room, Anne and I arranged furniture and clothing more conveniently. Nursing supplies were set on top of the dresser, or inside the drawers. Everything lay at my fingertips, just as any nurse would want.

"What about towels?" Anne asked, adjusting the lamp on the bed table. "Do you need a few more in here?"

But simultaneous ringing bells interrupted my response. Anne rushed to answer the front door, and I dashed into Dad's room to pick up the phone. The next sound I heard were male voices and clomping feet down the hallway. I peeked from the doorway and waved to my brothers-in-law, Larry and Randy, who were carrying the hospital bed. *Thank God!*

By the end of the brief telephone conversation, the original bed had been removed and the new one set into place. I eyed it nostalgically through the doorway, remembering another time. Wasn't it just yesterday that I had helped to haul each bed component down the monastery corridor? We leaned each section against the storage room wall and covered them with sturdy plastic. Though a weighty chore, it was equally gratitude-laden. *Someday it will serve a good purpose,* I remembered thinking. But no one could have imagined the actual outcome. Certainly not me.

I selected extra-long sheets for the hospital bed and tucked in the corners. I used the same blankets as before, but chose a different white bedspread this time. *Lighter weight. Much cooler.* I tugged on the sides, smoothing out the wrinkles. *Good. Now, time to get Mom.*

Her eyes were half closed as I approached her in the kitchen. Stoic, she was listening to Larry and Randy who recounted their monastery adventure.

"The nuns were great!" Randy said. "The whole community was out there helping."

"See, everyone loves you, Mom." I laid my hand on her shoulder.

"That's very nice. But could you put me back down?"

Her eyes were already shut as we tottered through the awkward transfer. Sinking onto the new mattress, she sighed, saying, "Oh, that's nice. Soft."

The bed motor hummed quietly as I operated the remote control and raised the head of the bed. No more would Mom suffer, lying unbearably prone all night. She was content and didn't notice when I left the room.

Afterward, I dashed up and down the stairs doing kitchen and laundry chores. All the while I kept an ear out for my sister Angie and her five young children who would soon visit us. Before long they arrived, announced by the familiar pitter-patter of small feet approaching the back doorway. From my vantage point at the kitchen sink, I watched as each child furtively filed in, obviously coached by "Mama" to keep the noise down.

Two-year-old Madeline was first. With index finger

poised to her lips, she strode toward me and dispatched her whispered order. "Shhhh! Gwam is asweep!" Rising on tiptoe, she spun around and crept stealthily down the hallway toward "Gram's" room.

Gram wasn't asleep, though. Before long we had all gathered at her side. She was happy to see the children, Hannah, Claire, Raphael, Madeline, and tiny Grace, whom Angie cradled in her arms. Mom lovingly took their hands and greeted each by name. But no one spoke. Stunned, only silent stares followed.

Blessed Mother, help them.

The stark atmosphere intensified as I pushed the wheelchair toward the bed and asked the children to step aside in the cramped space. "I have to get Gram up now," I explained. "A nurse is coming soon, and Gram needs to wait for him in the kitchen."

I reached under Mom's shoulders to lift her, which prompted four-year-old Raphael to finally speak. "Why can't she get up herself?"

"Because her leg won't work anymore." I turned and faced him. "She needs my help."

Silence.

In the next instant, Angie said, "Okay, kids, let's go. Gram needs to be with Jenny for awhile."

Mom felt badly. Once we were alone, she said, "They're afraid of me. It's hard for them."

"Yes." *It's hard for all of us.*

The nurse arrived and Dad led him into the kitchen where everyone was waiting. He took a seat next to Mom at the kitchen table and immediately set into business, asking questions.

"What medications are you taking, Agatha?" He inscribed the names into his notebook.

Looking at me, he asked, "Do you have one of these?" He reached into his bag and lifted out a plastic, seven-day pill container. I had never seen one.

I smiled. "No, but it would be very helpful to have."

He handed it to me.

There were more questions, more forms to fill out, followed by more questions. As before, the children observed in unbroken silence.

Again, it was perceptive Raphael, sitting next to me on the couch, who finally whispered, "Is he gonna fix Gram?"

"He's going to help make her feel better," I answered, not daring to show my disappointment. Promising a cure, I knew, was pointless.

Two weeks later, a coloring crayon picture of our house arrived in the mail, drawn by Raphael. It sported a square frame, a center-front door, two windows flanking, and a cozy, smoke-puffing chimney atop a triangle roof. Two pink daisies graced a soil-less garden and a smiling sun shone brilliantly in a white sky. In the lower right corner Gram was seated in the wheelchair, steering toward the house. As if communicating Raphael's thoughts, the picture seemed to conclude: "Gram will be in her wheelchair for a very long time."

Before leaving, the nurse asked to see a transfer. For the first time, I felt confident and moved smoothly through each step of the process. As I let Mom back down onto the bed, my larger than usual audience broke into applause, and Mom added her own vote of approval. "That was good."

Before the next appointment, I ran an errand down at the local hardware store. The idea was to find a piece of wood to attach to the end of Mom's bed. The blankets, I hoped, would flow over the top of it and create a weightless canopy above her feet. I spotted plywood pieces just inside the store entry. "On sale" the sign read over the large bin. Fishing through the pile, I selected a thin board and carried it to the clerk who cut it to size. At home, I padded the rough edges with foam rubber, covered it with an old flowered sheet, and vertically secured it in place.

I stepped back and studied the curious tower. "Definitely a homemade job."

But Mom was pleased and wriggled her toes to prove it.

Many times during these first harrowing days, I recalled my Carmelite years. In a real way I could not have cared for my mother without that experience. From the day I entered the monastery, not only did a life of contemplative prayer greet me, but also a brand new world of geriatric care. As a 23-year-old violinist, just a year out of college, it was at best a shock—no honeymoon. Love and its challenges were immediately set before me. Two of the elderly nuns had Alzheimer's disease. Others in the community needed special assistance. Gradually, by giving myself to prayer and the daily life, the experience unfolded as an invaluable gift. I grew to love caring for the sick, aged, and dying. *For the homebound and those who care for them,* I so often prayed. My petition had now reached into my own home, and I realized my mother and I were the team.

A physical therapist arrived in the late afternoon. Friendly and professional, she put Mom completely at ease. She began with exercises from the hospital, then promised to add new ones. That perked Mom up, who lay dressed in her knits on top of the bed. To her, any advancement in therapy meant more hope for recovery. Especially on the left side.

"How's that?" she asked, attempting to bend the left knee up a fraction of an inch more from the mattress. She grunted, pursing her lips from the effort. "Do you think it's getting any better?"

As with other therapists, the PT responded vaguely. She hoped her stock "You're-doing-very-well-Agatha" reply would suffice. But Mom was not convinced. Later, after failing to complete a particularly difficult movement, she looked directly at the therapist and posed the inevitable question. "Will I walk again?"

The PT hesitated.

Mom flashed a look toward me, which pleaded for hope.

She won't take "No" for an answer. Maybe that "dead area" in her brain that everyone keeps talking about will never recover. They told us that dead nerves have to find new pathways—or something like that. Is that what all of this therapy is for? Perhaps walking again is too much to hope for. Oh, God, help us to accept reality.

"I can't say for sure, Agatha," the therapist finally said, breaking the silence. "It's too soon to tell. Why don't we just call it a day?"

"Okay," Mom said, though disappointed. Reaching for her rosary, she lifted it from the bed table and began to pray.

The PT asked, "Can you take me to see the bathrooms now?"

I led her to the shower in Dad's room where she examined the shower bench. Satisfied, she followed me to the blue-tiled bathroom directly across from Mom's room and viewed the impractical design. The shower, set into an arty, sunken sort of bathtub, was accessible by two steps—impossible for Mom to use. The toilet, narrowly situated behind the door, was no better—a rehab nightmare. It didn't take long before the PT agreed that we had already worked out the best solutions.

"Just stick with the other shower," she said. "And keep using the commode."

Before leaving, she asked to see a transfer, scrutinizing each step. When Mom was seated again, the PT chuckled, saying, "Well, that was kind of a nice dance!" She scribbled something into her notes, looking up. "And I don't think I've ever seen anything quite like it before."

Choreographed or not, apparently our little "pas de deux" was working well. Pleased, the PT informed us to expect another therapist the next day. "He'll be a substitute in my place."

"Oh?" Mom's face fell. With so many therapists coming and going these days, she preferred consistency.

"Well, maybe he'll be just as good," I said, taking her hand after the PT had left.

"Yes, maybe," Mom returned, pensive.

Bedtime preparations began early, immediately following dinner. But unlike the night before, Mom felt strong and was able to stand at the sink to wash.

I used the commode to transport her into the bathroom. Seated in front of the sink, she grasped the commode's steel arm rest and prepared to push off. Standing at her left, I reached around her shoulders and lifted her to her feet. She paused, finding her balance, leaning heavily against the ceramic ledge.

"It feels so good to do something at least somewhat normally," she said, admiring her erect posture in the mirror.

But things were far from normal. Her left arm dangled, squeezed between her body and the hard ledge. I lifted it away, laying the palm flat down on the sink ledge. I never released my hold from around her shoulders. One-handedly I dampened the cloth under the water, studying Mom's face in the mirror. Though lined with wrinkles, she retained her beauty. Then another memory returned, triggered as she lifted the washcloth and began to wash her face.

As a child, I also stood at Mom's left, spellbound by her beauty. There, standing in front of the large mirrored dresser in her bedroom, she groomed herself for special occasions. Fragrant perfume wafted from inside the top dresser drawer, and my 5-year-old curiosity sizzled as I peeked inside, watching her select sparkly treasures from inside her rose-colored jewelry box. She combed and styled her dark brunette hair, tucking it up in a stylish roll, then secured it in place with a lovely pin. By the time she powdered over her gracefully defined facial features and smoothed on a glossy red lipstick, in my adoring eyes she was the vision of a queen.

"There!" Mom said, swatting the washcloth aside on the counter. She clung to the ledge, struggling for balance. "I need to get down."

I pleaded. "Just another minute, Mom. Can you do it? We need to brush your teeth."

She sighed. "Okay."

Back in her room, she settled into the hospital bed and operated the remote control. She snapped off the lamp switch and fingered over the table for her rosary. "I found it," she said, holding it up.

I turned, reminding her, "Ring if you need me. Promise?"

"Yes," she said, closing her eyes. "Goodnight, Little One. I love you. Thank you for everything."

Her peaceful words settled within, comforting my otherwise exhausted spirit as I left her room and walked down the hallway. Physically, I was keeping on top of things, but emotionally I felt ready to crumble. Tears found an outlet in prayer later that night as I realized, more than anything, I feared that Mom would die. *Not yet*, I prayed. *Please, not yet.*

But she was still close, and soon the bell rang.

"Could you pick up my rosary?" she asked, as I walked into her darkened room. Looking toward the lowered side bar of the hospital bed, she pointed. "It dropped."

"Probably caught on the rail." I walked around to the other side of the bed and stooped, freeing the snared rosary. I handed it back. "Sleep well now."

I walked down into the living room and settled in for the night. The day would surely come when I would no longer enjoy my mother's physical presence. But for now, I was grateful, and prayed to meet the next day's challenge.

The Third Day

The name of the feast day popped into my head as I awoke the next morning: *All Saints.* As if on cue, the Beatitudes began to speak within: "Blessed are you who are poor . . . Blessed you who are now weeping, for you will laugh." (Luke 6:20–21, Revised New Testament NAB) But Mom and I hadn't shared a laugh since she returned home. I climbed from the sleeping bag and pictured her helpless figure in bed, immobile. *Things are so serious . . . constant stress . . . emergencies . . . enormous adjustments. How can we laugh?* I turned to the Holy Spirit and prayed, *Please, grant us the gift of joy.*

I sat down on the living room rug to begin my exercises and reviewed the day's agenda. *Fewer visitors . . . somewhat of a help. But there will be unknown challenges.* I never knew what to expect. The trickiest consideration would come in the evening, when I was scheduled to attend an orchestra rehearsal at Seattle's St. James Cathedral. As a returning professional violinist in the area, I welcomed the opportunity but weighed our new circumstances. *Will Mom be all right while I'm gone? Maybe she'll need the commode . . . or be afraid without me. Maybe I should stay home.*

I lifted my arms high over my head and slowly bent forward. Touching my forehead to my extended straight legs, toes pointed, I breathed in deeply, then out, holding the soles of my feet for several seconds. Slowly I rose and straightened again, checking my inner barometer. *Steady . . . okay, go to the rehearsal as planned.*

Mom was awake when I checked on her after breakfast. Unusually energetic, she could hardly wait to show me something as she held up her left hand in her right. "Look, Jenny! I can move these two fingers a little."

Intrigued, I bent nearer and examined the fourth and little finger of her left hand, which were both curling and uncurling upon command. "That's great, Mom." But secretly I questioned the sudden spurt of movement. *Is this only temporary? She'll be disappointed if it doesn't stick.*

Dad joined us a few minutes later and Mom repeated her happy discovery for him. "That's wonderful, honey," he said, bending to view the fingers more closely.

She continued to prompt them while I dressed her. To her, the simple exercise was a challenging feat—an athletic undertaking. But when the effort grew labored and the fingers failed to respond, she stopped, crestfallen. "They won't move anymore. I guess I overdid it. I wish I could do more. I just don't know why I get so tired." She stroked her hand, staring at the fingers, returned to their curled, rigid state.

"Don't be so hard on yourself, Mom." I pulled a white sweatshirt over her head and guided the dead hand through the sleeve. "Rest is important, too, you know."

At breakfast, she turned on the TV to watch the news. I continued doing chores, keeping an eye on her from afar. *Is she eating?* Peeking around the corner, I checked for evidence. *No.* Entirely engrossed in the engaging world reports, she was oblivious to any food in front of her.

"Please, finish eating, Mom." I set my stack of folded laundry on the couch and pointed to the Shredded Wheat growing soggier by the second in her bowl.

Like a robot, she lifted the spoon, though without diverting her fascinated gaze from the screen. One mouthful, then she stopped.

"Congress today announced . . ."

The spoon slid back into the bowl.

A few minutes later, I pleaded, "Mom, please take another bite. You need to eat. Don't you understand? You need the calories."

"Stop nagging me!" she shot back, staring at the screen.

I knew I was nagging, but she needed the nourishment, so I tried another tactic. Sitting beside her, I picked up the spoon and wordlessly coaxed in the next mouthful.

"But the president plans to veto the measure . . ."

It worked. Like two runners handing off a baton in a relay race, Mom finally took to the rhythm and accepted the spoon. Eyes still glued to the TV, she finished feeding herself.

In the afternoon my sister Becky stopped by to visit. She offered to cut Mom's hair, quickly devising a makeshift salon in her room. While Mom sat in the wheelchair, Becky cut open a black lawn-and-leaf bag and wrapped it around her like a huge salon cape. When the haircut was finished, Mom viewed her shorter bob through a handheld mirror. Satisfied, she waited as I adjusted a pink knit headband around her ears.

"Perfect," she said.

"You look pretty tired, though." I helped her to

stand, then transferred her back into bed, pulling up the bedspread. "The new PT will be here in a little while. Do you still want to go through with this?"

"I have to." She reached for her water cup. "It's my only hope to walk again. Maybe he'll be able to help me."

At 4 o'clock the doorbell rang. Finished with a quick practice session on the violin, I set my instrument down and ran from the living room to check on Mom. She was barely awake.

"Just let him in," she said, giving a short wave of her hand. She struggled to keep her eyes open. "I'll be fine."

I greeted the young man in the front hallway and we exchanged the usual introductions. I was just about to escort him into Mom's room—secretly hoping we could bypass bathroom tours this time—when he drew close to my face, and said, "Now, I'd like to see the shower and the toilet."

Groan.

Leading him into the first bathroom, I showed him the shower bench and explained that everything had been worked out with the other therapists. Unconvinced, he inquired into other options. When I escorted him to the bathroom outside of Mom's room, he glanced only briefly at its tiered layout before launching into his plan—something about filling in the sunken bathtub with cement and installing a special ramp and rail. When he got to the part about "just wheeling her over the top," I had heard enough.

I interrupted. "Excuse me, but if you don't mind, this is much too complicated. We're not prepared to think in these terms yet. No one knows exactly how Mom's recovery will go. Maybe she'll walk again."

He stared, his next words caught in his throat.

I continued. "The other shower will be fine. Would you like to meet my mother now?"

He consented.

Leading him to her room, I introduced Mom to him. Then he looked at me and asked to see a transfer. Again, I explained that a good method had already been worked out with the other therapists. "Besides, Mom is very tired. She can't get up to do this right now."

Determined, he persisted, forcing a strained smile. "Then why don't you just sit down and I'll demonstrate on you."

I negotiated, straight-faced. "I don't see how that will do any good. I'm much lighter than she is. It's unrealistic. Please—"

But he pushed onward. "Well, may I just show you once?"

I sighed. "Okay, once." Reluctantly, I sat down in the wheelchair. *Just get it over with.* I stared up at him. "Now what do I do?"

Quickly, he bent forward and reached around the back of my hips. "This will be personal. Do you mind?"

I did, but before I could respond, he had pulled me to my feet where I stood, annoyed at his manner and unimpressed by his system. I stepped back. "I doubt I could lift Mom that way. She's too heavy and doesn't have enough power to help."

"Well, at least you can try, can't you?" he asked, his voice rising.

"I just don't—"

"Are we going to start the exercises now?" Mom chimed in, suddenly cheerful as she came to my rescue.

Caught off guard, the therapist turned toward her, and stuttered, "All . . . all right." Then, regrouping, he looked at me again and slowly held up his right index finger. He directed, "Now, I need an ice cube."

"An ice cube?"

"Yes, and a paper towel."

"Right . . ."

Incredulous, I walked to the kitchen and opened the freezer door. Selecting one very cold ice cube from the tray, I wondered what all of this could possibly be leading to. *Mom has worked with 14 doctors since the stroke. Specialists, we were told, every one. Is the matter now to be resolved with a puny ice cube? Please!* I opened the cupboard door below the sink and tore a paper towel from the roll.

Returning to Mom's room, I handed the ice cube to the therapist who rolled up Mom's pant leg to the knee and described how he would slide the frozen chip up and down her shin. "Like this," he said, demonstrating the ridiculous technique with sweeping gestures in the air. This, he explained, would fire the brain, somehow kicking the leg back into motion. A miracle!

And so he began, directing Mom to simultaneously pull her knee up as far as possible. Not surprisingly, nothing happened. All she managed was her usual struggle for a few inches of height.

Finally, the therapist asked, "Do you feel anything yet?"

"Yes, it's cold!" Mom said, helplessly batting his hand away.

Instantly, he stopped and dabbed the numbed limb with the paper towel.

Just then, Dad walked through the doorway and

informed me I had a phone call. Leaving to answer it, I glanced once more over my shoulder. But this time the PT was lifting the waistband of Mom's pants and following down inside with the ice cube. *Now what?* Knowing she was safe with Dad, I left.

But when I returned, Mom was wild-eyed. As if her frozen predicament had not been enough, she was now caught in the midst of a lecture—trapped!—listening as the therapist rambled on and on, explicating various theories of therapy. Things were getting nowhere.

Unable to bear it any longer, she suddenly forced a smile, reached up, and shook his hand in mid-sentence. "Thank you very much, good-bye!"

Stunned, he stopped, releasing her hand. Then, collecting his things, he attempted a less-than-successful farewell. Turning, he left without further fanfare.

Time was extremely short afterward, so we didn't discuss anything of the fiasco. I only had time to quickly prepare dinner and arrange things so that Mom would be comfortable until I returned home from rehearsal.

"Just enjoy yourself," she kept saying, kindly looking up from her pillow as I scuttled around the room. She pulled the blanket up herself, using a newly attached drawstring pinned to the blanket hem. Stuffing the end into a plastic towel holder taped to the side of the bed table, she reassured me, "Your father and I will be fine."

The drive down to the cathedral helped to shift my thoughts to musical matters. We would perform Mozart's "Requiem" the next evening on the feast of All Souls. The last time I performed Mozart's masterpiece was in my teens. But that was long ago and the present experience felt like a fresh beginning.

I entered the cathedral, enveloped by the vast, sacred space, and set my violin case down in a pew. Looking up, I recognized a friend from my past, who approached and greeted me. Self-conscious at first, I soon relaxed and chatted with several other friends who also gathered around and inquired about Mom. "How is she?" The news had traveled fast.

"As well as can be expected," I told them. "But it's very difficult."

I tried to set "Mom" thoughts aside as I took my seat in the orchestra and drew my bow on the downbeat. Caregiving distractions meandered in between reading notes on the page, along with other interjections—"You were a nun, weren't you?" my unfamiliar stand partner asked during a rest. But I was getting used to that, and kept on, grateful for the musical respite.

The next evening, following the performance, I was surprised to see the head nurse from the hospital, who came up and greeted me. We stood beside orchestra chairs and I recounted our hair-raising return from the hospital. I explained to her that it was doubly difficult for us, because of our lack of preparation from the hospital staff.

She listened carefully, grateful to have the information for future patients and their families. Taking my hand, she encouraged me. "Just don't lose your confidence with the transfers."

"No, I won't."

We parted on good terms.

When I returned home after the concert, Mom was asleep. Taking the opportunity to get an earlier start on rest myself, I climbed into my sack and instantly dozed off. An hour later, the bell rang.

"How did it go?" Mom asked, as I padded to her side in slippered feet.

"Fine. But I want to hear about you. Were there any problems while I was gone?"

"No, not a thing," she said, content. "Everything went well. But I need a clean diaper. Could you help me, please?"

I thought I must by sleepy, or perhaps just imagining things. But as I changed her diaper, everything suddenly seemed relaxed, without a trace of tension. *Maybe we're finally getting used to this.* I walked to the foot of the bed and adjusted the blankets. Then, looking up at Mom, I saw her peering at me with a twinkle in her eye and a mischievous grin on her face. I hadn't seen that in awhile.

"What are you smiling about?" I asked.

"I don't know about that guy today," she said, giggling as her grin widened.

"What guy?" I searched my memory, trying to sort out the array of so many new faces.

She giggled some more. "You know, Ice Cube."

At the sound of the perfectly selected name, the afternoon ordeal returned and we burst into laughter. Peals of it!

"What was he doing in your pants with that ice cube?" I asked, relieved to finally solve the puzzle.

"He said he needed to stimulate some kind of a nerve in the top of the leg. I told him it was cold!"

As our laughter increased, I couldn't help noticing the increased volume in Mom's voice, a total contrast to her softer tone after the stroke. Then I sensed something deeper, more than mere fun for Mom. It seemed the moment had also become an immense emotional release, as if the burden of her whole life was pouring out in laughter. Thinking she might prefer solitude to just "laugh it out," so to speak, I stepped into the hallway and quietly closed the door behind me. Waiting, I took in the full import of her ongoing, uproarious "song."

When at last it simmered to intermittent chuckles, I rejoined her at bedside, and asked, "Feeling better?"

"Yes," she said, teary with joy as she wiped her eyes. "But you have to understand, honey, I don't have any defenses left."

What surprising words to hear from my crippled, elderly mother in the middle of the night. Delighted, I leaned over and wrapped her in a hug. "Well, that's awfully nice, Mom. You're about the luckiest person in the world."

Holding her for another moment, she quieted, then closed her eyes. Knowing she was peaceful, I left.

Back in my corner, I reflected on our first days, which now seemed like a foundational triptych. Establishing Mom's home care had been much more difficult than expected, but the third day had resolved in surprising joy. I heard the promise of Jesus now, as it filtered through my mind again," . . . you will laugh." *Yes, we will continue, rejoicing and full of gladness.*

The Way of Friends

I pulled off the wet flannel draw sheet from Mom's bed and stuffed it into the green plastic waste can—the "hamper"—designated as such in the scuffle of setting up her room. Soon, I would have to reapply duct tape around the rim, though; the cracks were spreading. Mom didn't mind. She had always been content with a simple lifestyle.

"When your father and I first started out," she told me, "we didn't have any money, so I made all of Mark's baby clothes by hand and used orange crates for dresser drawers."

That was in 1946.

"Was it hard?" I asked.

"No," she replied, beaming. "We were just so happy."

As Mom shared more of these vignettes, I loved to hear them.

I grasped the waste can and carried it down to the laundry room. Meanwhile, Mom sat in the kitchen, eating breakfast. The familiar sound of the *Today Show* filled the background. After more than a week into our new endeavor, we were beginning to settle into a routine.

I tossed the billowy load into the washing machine and recalled the shower the evening before. It was just before bedtime and, under the circumstances, a "big deal."

Not only had we overcome the final obstacle in facilitating Mom's care at home, but for me, the time also afforded a new insight into the Gospel: Jesus' example of humble service. Caring for Mom would often provide that.

The bed blankets were neatly doubled back and draped over the footboard. I laid everything we would need on top of the exposed sheets: clean nightie, new diaper, comb, portable hair dryer, and a well-worn, brown neck scapular of Our Lady of Mt. Carmel. Each item was lined up in a particular order and, though ordinary, appeared special to me because my mother was so special.

The commode lacked a footrest, so I wheeled Mom backward from her room, passing through Dad's room to reach the shower. Dressed in a long-sleeved pink nightie, her toes lightly skimmed the floor, hugged by fuzzy blue footies.

"Oh, this will feel nice," she said, her spirits lifting as she glided closer to the goal.

But my sentiments differed. Anticipating the first transfer over a tile floor, the sight of the small floor mat in front of the shower offered no comfort. I concentrated, trying to keep focused.

I parked Mom alongside the shower and mustered up my courage. Stooping, I clamped down on the noisy commode brakes—Clunk! Clunk!—then straightened and buckled her transfer belt. I checked and rechecked the fitting. *Snug enough? I think so . . . no, a little more.* I pulled. *Please, don't let me drop her.*

Ready, I reached under her arms and lifted her, eyeing the remaining breach between the shower ledge and the bench. "Don't be alarmed," I told Mom, tightening my hold as we stepped twice, pivoting into position. "I can't let go of you, so I'll have to push against your thighs to scoot your hips the rest of the way onto the bench. Understand? You can't cross the gap on your own."

"Got it," Mom said, maintaining her single-armed clutch around me. "Go ahead."

One firm nudge was all it took. As Mom's hips squarely met the unseen bench behind her, she loosened her grasp, and said, "That was good!" She looked more like a little girl ready for a tea party now.

Looking to her right, she reached for the specially installed stainless steel handrail affixed to the shower wall. Holding onto it, she watched as I gathered her legs from under the knees and lifted them into the shower.

She's in! Pulling off my socks, I rolled up my sweatpants and shirt sleeves. I pulled my hair back into a ponytail and removed Mom's gown. Laying it on the sink ledge, I climbed into the shower. For the first time, I noticed light blue decorations on the tile. "Huh, daisy things." I turned and faced Mom from my snug corner. Tucked in on her right, there was just enough room for the two of us.

She chuckled. "It's a good thing you're not any bigger." Reaching across her tummy, she tried to pull the clear plastic curtain closed, but I finished the task, too much of a reach for her.

Swoosh! On went the water, but without touching Mom yet. I was holding the portable hose to the side and adjusted the temperature. As I lifted the nozzle, the first splash spilled down her back.

She protested, jerking forward with surprising energy. "It's too hot!"

"Sorry." I pulled the hose away and adjusted the temperature. "Better?"

"No!" she said, lurching forward again. "Now it's too cold!"

"Then I guess that makes you Baby Bear, and me Goldilocks, right?"

We laughed.

Appropriately, the third attempt was "just right." Mom visibly relaxed under the water's warm massage and moved much more naturally than I had seen since the stroke. Her motions were relaxed, flowing with a casual freedom. She enjoyed independently rubbing the soapy washcloth around her body, then handed me the cloth when areas were out of her reach.

Grasping the back bar of the bench for balance, I bent and scrubbed her feet.

She resisted, playfully kicking my hand away. "It tickles."

"Even before I've touched you?" I paused, joining her laughter from my upside-down perspective.

From the bedroom, Dad noticed our mirth and added to the fun. "What are you two girls laughing about?"

Perhaps Mom and I should have been bitter, or depressed. But to the contrary we were happy, immersed in a brand new relationship, more like sisters.

I lifted the nozzle over her head. "Here goes." The warm stream rushed like a waterfall and peeled the hair flat against her face. "You look like Mary and I used to," I said, smiling at the childhood memory with my next oldest sister. "Remember when you gave us baths together?"

In those days, Mary and I sat waist-deep in the warm water of our old-fashioned footed bathtub. Mom, dressed in a cotton housedress, knelt at the side of the tub and scrubbed bargain-buy shampoo into our hair. She pressed tiny strokes behind our ear lobes, saying, "You need to get all the way behind the ears," and often added her favorite adage: "A mother has to teach her children."

When the time came for the hair rinse, Mary and I held our breath, watching as Mom lifted the orange rubber hose over our heads. Quickly, we plugged our noses and snapped our eyes shut to avoid the soapy sting.

Now, with her nose also pinched closed and her eyes squeezed shut, Mom appeared the same to me, only I held the hose and for a very different reason.

I turned off the water and reached for the towel, laid on the mat just outside the curtain. I moved swiftly, never knowing when Mom's energy might drain.

"Oh, it's cold," she said, feeling the chilly air as the curtain opened. Quickly, she drew her right arm in front of her, attempting to guard her wet skin; the slightest breeze was enough to trigger a goose-bump eruption.

I unfurled the white towel and squeezed her hair dry with one end, while she buffed the lower part of her body with the other. What she couldn't manage, she patiently waited for me to complete.

"Let's do the standing now," I said, slinging the towel over my right shoulder as I prepared to lift her. "I need to dry the back of you, Mom." Then I stopped.

"Just a second," she said, lifting her left hand with her right.

What's she up to now? Doesn't she know her arm can't help?

Intent, she struggled to hook the crippled fingers over the handrail in front of her.

"What are you doing, Mom?" I already knew the

answer, but controlled my urge to snap. *This will never work!*

"I want to help with the standing," she said, determined as she reexamined each finger. She braced her right palm against the bench and gave the signal. "Okay, I'm ready."

But I wasn't. Aware of the futility, I hesitated. *Should I stop her?*

"No," came the inward answer.

My frustration, I realized, was not the point. At that moment, Mom needed to discover her own limits.

Resigned, I began to lift her. Helping, she pushed off from the bench. But her attempt failed miserably and the powerless fingers slid from the rail, dropping the arm flaccidly to her side again.

"Oh, that darn arm!" she sighed, defeated.

"The right works fine." I choked back my disappointment, attempting to downplay the incident. "You did the best you could."

We proceeded in silence as I dried the back of her body. When she was seated again, I slipped her gown on and stepped from the shower. I pulled the commode into place, set the brakes, swiveled her legs over the ledge, and knelt at her feet to dry them. Then everything changed. Suddenly, I felt as if we were reenacting the washing-of-the-feet episode from the Gospel, when Jesus washed his disciple's feet. At the same moment, the Master's words came to mind: " . . . as I have done for you, so you should also do." (John 19:27, Revised New Testament NAB)

Inspired, I lifted Mom's long feet, markedly cooler and bluish in color from poor circulation, and began to dry them. My cross, I understood, was to witness her daily, countless limitations. But I also realized that I needed to be more patient, accepting her as she was. *How would I feel in the same situation?* Mom, like me, needed merciful love.

"Now, for the ten tiny toes," I said, prepared for the sobering task of drying in between them; I knew Mom would hate that.

Wincing, she pleaded, "Watch that toe!" as I worked the thick terry cloth in between the first two digits.

I continued, doggedly anchoring her right heel in my hands. She resisted, pulling back.

"Now, all I have to do is put your footies on," I said, picking up the first one from the floor. I struggled to inch the cotton spandex over her clammy skin, complicated by bunions, which protruded from both feet.

Finished, I sat back on my heels to rest and noted the precious picture of Mom's sweet face, framed by wet, loosely tangled hair. Seeing her look at me with so much love, I wondered, *Is it Mom or Jesus?*

The commode wheels squeaked as I guided her back to her room. Once seated alongside the bed, she snatched up the hairdryer lying on the mattress and switched it on. She piloted the warm air stream all around her wet hair, as I stood behind and eased out the tangles, separating the blowing strands between my fingers. When her hair was dry again, I called out over the loud motor, "Done!"

She flipped off the switch and laid the hairdryer down. In the same motion, she asked for baby powder. "I just love the smell."

I opened the cupboard door in the bathroom and located the small bottle on the top shelf. Carrying it back to Mom, she smiled and sprinkled it lightly over her chest. As she patted the fragrant powder into her skin, she reminisced:

"When I was a little girl, my mother always used baby powder after a baby was born. I just loved having new babies in the house."

I lifted her nightie from the mattress and guided her left arm through the sleeve. Her gaze followed to the right sleeve and she mechanically reached through the opening. Still smiling, she continued to describe her youngest sister's arrival.

"I remember the day that Mother brought Carolyn home—it was the first day of spring—and I smelled baby powder in the house. I was so happy. I went for a walk outside and met the parish priest along the way. I said to him, 'Father, isn't it wonderful? It's the first day of spring, and I have a new baby sister!'"

Absorbed in her childhood account, I thirsted to hear more. But it wasn't to be that night. Mom suddenly bowed her head, exhausted.

"Maybe you could tell me more some other time." Quickly, I stepped in front of the wheelchair and reached under her arms to begin the transfer. "Up now, before you lose your strength."

A few mornings later, hearing the bell, I left the half-filled pillbox on the kitchen counter and walked down the hallway to answer it. I thought, *Mom probably needs the commode.* Reaching her side I was taken aback when she looked up, and asked, instead, "Jenny, do you think it would be good for me to take Tylenol now or later?"

Her open, childlike gaze was filled with trust, as if she was expecting an answer from "Mommy." *Does she really think of me that way?* Still, as her daughter, I teased, "You always made decisions like that for yourself, Mom. The Tylenol bottle is right next to you on the table." I pointed to the jumbo-size plastic container, which was also propping up a small picture of Jesus. "Wasn't I the one who always asked you those kinds of questions?"

But two mornings later, she revealed the full extent of her trust. As I helped her onto the commode, then back into bed, she looked at me, and confided, "You're my best friend."

Her words, quietly spoken, resounded all through me. *Best friend!* From the onset of her care, even more than a nurse, I had prayed that Mom would trust me as a friend, comfortable to share every moment of her journey with me. My prayer had now been granted and I took her hand.

"When you said you would take care of me that first day in the kitchen," she explained, "I felt safe, because I knew you had been through a lot and would understand."

"I do understand," I assured her, "and you're my best friend, too."

It was a turning point. Acknowledging our special friendship, our bond was strengthened. But challenges remained. For me, friendship meant the hour by hour, minute by minute commitment of being there for Mom, no matter what. Our elbows rubbed constantly, from one transfer to the next, one meal to another, the next diaper change, clothing change, and shower.

But most of all, it was the bell, that constant little ding-dinging, which increasingly rattled my nerves over the course of the next few months. Yet again hearing it for the sixth time one night, I stepped from my sleeping bag, exhausted, convinced I had no resources of patience left. Certainly, I gave no thought to prayer as I dragged myself down the hallway, feeling anger well to the surface. When I entered Mom's room, I stood by her bed, my long, disheveled hair appropriately matching my inner disorder, and burst into tears. "What do you want now?" Immediately, a rush of guilt followed. *How can I be so awful?* I covered my face with my hands. *Can I truly call myself Mom's friend?* I was finally praying.

When I looked up again, she was serene, and smiled, saying, "Oh dear, honey. You're behaving just like a new mother."

Gathering my senses, I realized she was right. Any new mother or caregiver would understand that. And who, better than my own mother, a nurturer of ten and champion of late-night feedings? Her compassion at that moment was an experience of God's friendship—she loved me at my worst.

Softly, she said, "You'll be fine, Jenny. I know you will."

But trials continued. Repeating a similar scenario several weeks later, I again found myself on "midnight knees," uttering words of repentance. But Mom helped to heal my ruffled spirit, again admitting her own weakness. "Don't let it bother you, Little One. It took me years to get over resenting having to get up with all of you in the night."

Years! If Mom, with all of her talent, faith, and goodwill had struggled, perhaps I could learn as well.

From then on, I gently prodded her to share more about her experience as a mother.

"Just what was it like to raise so many children?"
I asked, seated one afternoon on the chest at the foot of
her bed, my usual perch. One by one, I lifted diapers from
the large cardboard box at my feet and taped the sides
together; I filled a dresser drawer-full of them at a time.

"There were days when I could have sold all of you
for a nickel," she confessed, smiling. She offered a knowing look as I completed my diaper duty.

I tamped down on the plastic bulk and shoved the
door closed. "There."

"Thanks for doing that."

"Did you have any favorites?" I asked, continuing
the "interview" as I sat back down on the chest. "I mean,
among the children?"

"No, I loved you all."

Glowing, she reached for her left arm and lifted it
from beneath the bedspread. Overheated, the hand was
moist and she uncurled the fingers to cool them on top
of her tummy. Then she reached behind and slipped her
right palm beneath her head on the pillow. "It's so hard
not being able to change positions." She pulled her right
knee up beneath the covers, a minor relief.

I continued. "So, what was the hardest part about
raising children?"

"No gratitude," she replied, without hesitation.
"Children can be so selfish. They don't realize how much
you're giving to them. Everything is 'gimme, gimme.'
That's really hard on a parent."

"I wish I had been more grateful." I rolled my eyes,
shaking my head, reminded of my self-centered youth.

Mom smiled. "Don't think about it anymore. The
past is gone."

As the weeks unfolded, it became harder to watch Mom suffer, but I didn't always realize it. I tried to be strong and meet her daily needs, smiling through my tasks. But one morning, as I prepared to wash her, the mere sight of her helpless figure caught me off guard. Reality sank deeper, and I realized she couldn't do anything. I paused, imagining a future day, perhaps that very moment, when she would stand and walk again. But as usual, immobile, she waited for me to assist her. Filled with these thoughts, tears welled to the surface and I slunk down in the wheelchair behind me and let my emotions overflow. I didn't want to upset her, so stood to leave the room.

Then she spoke. "It's hard for you to see your mother like this."

I nodded, wiping my tears.

"Please, sit back down, then," she said, gesturing with her palm toward the wheelchair. "Let me tell you my own story."

Calmly, she began to describe the experience of caring for her own mother, Nellie, who was stricken with a blood clot in the lung at the young age of 38. For 13-year-old Agatha, who was the oldest of the family's four children, it was a sad and confusing time. Though ignorant of any kind of skilled nursing, she still agreed to be her mother's main caregiver at home.

"I didn't even know enough to give her a sponge bath," she admitted. "I wish I had known." Continuing, she described her two younger sisters, Shirley and Carolyn, who didn't want to believe that their mother would die. They spent the entire last evening of her life praying at her bedside. Nellie's final words to them were simply, "Always mind Dad and Agatha."

"What was it like when she finally died?" Standing, I walked to Mom's side, wanting to be nearer as she finished her gripping story.

"It was very sad," she said, peering up from eyes, which reflected the past's somber emotions. "My father, especially, was bereft. He used to sit by the stove every night for hours, not knowing how to reach out to any of us. It took him a long time to come out of it. I suffered more from seeing what he went through, than from anything else."

"You were so young. Did you have anyone to help you through your grief?"

"No. I cried myself to sleep every night for a year."

I paused, imagining the bleak scene: A lone, grieving teenager in a dark bedroom. The next part of the story seemed clearer, then. "You became the mother to your younger brother and sisters. Is that right?"

"I suppose I did," Mom responded, letting her gaze wander as she gathered more thoughts. Then looking at me again, she said, "But I don't know if I was much good at it. I didn't even know how to cook. One of the neighbor ladies had to teach me. I just did the best I could."

Bending, I embraced her. Like living out a vocation, Mom had accepted the challenges of motherhood from her earliest years. Bravely, she learned each lesson, but only in the process—no pre-made formulas.

"Maybe I'll get better at what I'm doing, too, Mom."

"You're doing a very good job."

"Thanks." I stood up straight, my burden lifted. "I love you."

"I know you do. But I've really got to get up now."

With a quick motion of her hand, she pulled back the bedspread, smiling again. "Should we start the washing now?"

"Right. Back on the job."

Also able to smile, I reached for the water basin, ready to care for my best friend.

Traveling Again

It was during her initial hospital stay after the stroke that Mom decided her traveling days were over.

"Now I won't be able to go anywhere," she said. "To Mass, out to dinner, or to concerts." Seated in the wheelchair, she stared vacantly out of the hospital window, unaffected by the panorama of autumn-leafed trees blazing in golds and reds on the crisp, sunny afternoon. Her normally rosy complexion had sallowed, offset by the pale, flimsy hospital gown that she wore. The ball of her right foot, encased in a thin, rubber-soled slipper, pushed repeatedly into the floor, generating even pulsations of movement. Rocking back and forth, she seemed to cradle her own frailty.

Will this be Mom's entire existence, rocking back and forth in a wheelchair?

"But that's not true, Agatha," Dad said, his strong voice slicing the dreariness and offering hope. He leaned forward in his chair and placed his large hand over hers. "Sure you'll be able to get out again, honey. We'll do all of those things together."

Mom turned slightly, restricted by her limited range of neck motion. "But I'm in a wheelchair, Bill. I'll just be a burden. No fun for you or Jenny, anymore."

It was my turn. "It won't be impossible, Mom.

There are lots of places that accommodate the disabled. At least we can try, can't we?"

No answer. Overwhelmed, she looked toward the window, unable to envision any horizon beyond the four walls of her sterile surroundings. Time and physical healing were necessary before any kind of traveling would appeal to her.

The first opportunity arose soon after, posed as a suggestion by a hospital therapist. "We're going to take you for a ride, Agatha," she announced, "so that you can see the possibilities of getting out a little. I'm sure you'll enjoy that. How about it?"

"All right," Mom said, though unenthusiastic.

Her reservation proved true. Riding in a specially equipped van for handicapped passengers, she was escorted to a scenic park on Lake Washington. The sunny October day was unusually warm, and everything seemed positive enough. But when Dad, her excursion partner, returned home later that afternoon, his report to me was bleak.

"It didn't go well," he said, dropping his car keys on top of the dresser in the hallway and walking into the kitchen. He sat down next to me at the table. "She didn't like the way they had her all strapped down in the van. She asked to return to the hospital immediately after we wheeled her out at the park. It was awful."

The next day I brought up the incident with Mom, urging her to try again. But her stance was irrevocable. "I hated it. I never want to go in the van again." Fixing her gaze on the partially drawn window curtain, she said, "Well, at least I have a nice house and a view at home."

Will Mom be a homebound prisoner for the rest of her

life? I struggled to accept the limited notion. *Can't she enjoy more than a view?*

Closing her eyes, she fell into a deep sleep. Feeling the need to also be in the quiet, I knelt, vigilant as a night watch beside her figure. The familiar contours of her face led like a pathway, and I soon found myself back at a favorite location, recalling the lovely setting of a beach.

As a child of six, I ambled with Mom along the rocky shore of Fort Flagler on the Olympic Peninsula, the scenic locale of the Seattle Youth Symphony's annual Marrowstone Music Festival. While Dad was occupied as the festival's music director and conductor, and my older siblings participated in the orchestra and chamber music groups, Mom and I spent private time together, often walking.

The beach, both rugged and serene, was strewn with jagged hunks of driftwood, embedded permanently against a scraggy, weather-beaten bluff. To the north, a lighthouse droned foghorn warnings on mist-laden days and nights, and to the south, an old wooden dock stretched out over the water. Silhouetted against the majestic peak of Mount Rainier in the distance, the little dock was a symbol of strength to me, bearing up in spite of powerful currents, which swirled beneath it.

As Mom and I continued to stroll, I collected handfuls of rocks and shells. At each find, I exclaimed, "Look at this!" and lofted each treasure high over my head for her careful examination. Whether sharing my fascination or not, she always responded enthusiastically, even after an already overabundant number of repetitions.

After playtime with my friends in the evening, I looked for Mom and usually found her sitting, recollected on the wooden steps of our primitive turn-of-the-century army bungalow. Dried grass and wild orange poppies adorned her surroundings, and her peaceful gaze held the panoramic view of the water in the distance. Seeing me approach, she invited me to sit beside her. Then she pulled me close, saying, "God loves you very much, and so do I."

When she returned home from the hospital, her surroundings were as predicted, "A nice house and a view." If not in bed, she sat near the kitchen window staring out over Lake Washington, or wheeled a few feet backward, where she watched TV from her favorite corner. If a suspenseful movie succeeded in captivating her interest for a few hours, the idea of venturing out to experience the world beyond did not.

I finally prodded her one afternoon from down the hallway. Carrying a stack of folded towels, I caught her eye during a TV commercial, and asked, "How about just wheeling around the driveway a few times, Mom? You don't even have to get in the car. I'll just put a coat over your shoulders and we'll be back in the house in a few minutes."

"Too much," was all she said, turning toward the TV again. Withdrawn into her protected world, she was satisfied.

But a week later, she surprised me by agreeing to visit Angie's family, the Russells. Feeling an unexpected boost of energy that morning, the prospect of getting in the car to see her grandchildren was a happy one.

My little red car idled in the carport, warming up as Dad and I fussed over Mom in the front hallway. Just to get her coat on required a team effort.

"Here, hold on," I said, helping her to stand from the wheelchair.

She stood, balanced against me for support.

Moving quickly, Dad guided her left arm through the coat sleeve, then yanked, straightening the twisted fabric from around her back and shoulders. Mildly successful, he walked to her right and held up the other sleeve. "Can you see it, honey?"

"No," she said, unable to turn her head. She leaned more heavily against me, releasing her grasp from around my shoulder. "But I can feel for the mark."

She was in.

Easing her down, I buttoned the coat. Dad lifted her foot onto the footrest and waited as I wrapped a white chiffon scarf over her head and tied it under her chin. "You don't mind the little hole in the corner, do you?"

"No, I'm used to it."

Dad opened the back door.

Taking in the first whiff of crisp air, Mom sighed. "Oh, that smells good. I forgot how wonderful fresh air is."

The wheelchair bumped over the aluminum door frame and I guided Mom to the car. Angling the wheelchair alongside the open passenger door, I helped her to stand.

Already, she was laughing. "Just like moving a sack of potatoes!"

I hoisted her down onto the car seat, but misjudged the momentum. Quickly, she slid from my grasp and toppled sideways.

"Sorry!" Also laughing, I loosened my grasp and

doubled over, laying my head on her shoulder. "This is too funny."

"I know," Mom said, her voice muffled as she dangled over the stick shift. She attempted to push herself up. "Could you help me, please?"

Used to our antics, Dad ignored the comedy and concentrated on wrangling the wheelchair into the trunk. Finished, he slammed the lid, then waited as I regained my composure and righted Mom. I popped the new handicapped decal into the glove compartment and snapped the door shut. "There." Our place in the traveling world of the disabled was now official.

We waved to Dad and set off. I stopped at the first street corner and readjusted Mom's left arm, supported for the ride in a sling.

"Just hold it here," I explained. "Like this . . . next to you." I adjusted her right arm, pinned under the seat belt.

Driving on, I listened as she reminisced about her days in the hospital, that traumatic time when life had so drastically changed. The medical staff, especially, left a lasting impression. She never tired of retelling the tales.

There was Prince, for instance, the ornery nurse.

"When Prince walked into the room," Mom said, chuckling, "it was like watching a big ship come over the horizon. She stood at the foot of my bed, glowering, put out if I asked her to do one more thing."

But like everyone else on the staff, Mom grew to love her very much.

"She (Prince) finally admitted one day that she didn't enjoy her work. But it was the only employment she could find. I really felt sorry for her."

I checked my wristwatch, aware of each passing second. *Her energy will be good for a little over an hour. Just enough time to visit with the Russells, then return home. She'll be tired, so I'd better not wear her out with more conversation.*

I didn't have to try. Mom had already tuned me out, silently focused on sights out the window.

We rounded the last street corner and arrived at the Russell's home. Eagerly the children bolted from the front door and pranced in bare feet over the gravel driveway. They waved, squealing, "Hi, Gram!"

I reached across Mom and rolled down the window.

"Hi, kids." Subdued, she smiled through the effort of turning her head. She looked toward the front door—so near. But today she wouldn't walk toward it as she had so many times in the past.

"We'll have a board for you to ramp up onto the porch next time," Angie said, reading Mom's thoughts as she stood by the car window, looking toward the door. "Please, come again. It's just one step up."

The children were more relaxed with Gram this time. Their words tripped over one another as they shared stories about school, projects, and pets. What Mom didn't realize was the joy she inspired, simply by her presence. To the grandchildren, Gram would always be special, disabled or not.

But after only a few minutes, she announced, "I've got to leave now, Jenny. Let's go." Bowing her head, she laid it in her palm. Looking up a moment later, she waved farewell, listening to the children who again exploded in squeals, jumping up and down.

"Did I do all right?" she asked, as I backed out of the driveway.

"You did great." Affectionately, I rubbed her cheek with the back of my hand. "See, Mom? You can get out a little."

"I guess I can."

The next outing occurred a few weeks later when outpatient therapy began at the hospital. The first appointment fell on a Tuesday morning in December, a heavy rain falling as we drove downtown. Turning into the uncovered parking lot, I pulled into a handicapped space and hung the decal on the rearview mirror. I handed Mom a small, maroon umbrella from the back seat, walked back to the trunk, and lifted out the wheelchair. I pushed it alongside Mom's open door and she popped open the umbrella, holding it over her head. I bent and swiveled her legs from the car.

"Please, hold the umbrella higher," I said, dodging the spokes as I reached under her arms. Concentrating, she lifted it higher as I pulled her to her feet. Letting her down into the chair, I guided her down the unfamiliar sidewalk and glanced toward the building's large, ground-floor windows. "This has to be the place."

Through the window, we could see a group of seniors hard at work in an aerobic class. Seated, they were all lifting arms and legs in unison. I made a sharp left turn down another sidewalk and steered toward the entrance. "You'll fit right in, Mom."

The automatic doors slid open and a large sign directed us straight ahead to the outpatient therapy department.

"Agatha Sokol is here for her appointment," I told the receptionist, as we arrived at the front desk.

The young woman peered over the top of her glasses, searching for Mom who was half hidden below the high counter. "Very well. Your therapist will be out shortly."

I looked around. *Mmm, new circumstances. Where to put Mom?* All of the roomy spots were taken, so I chose a space in front of the magazine table. *Not ideal, but the best I can do.* "Sorry about this, Mom." I slowly backed her in.

In the next instant, a gentleman stood and gingerly reached around her, attempting to lift a periodical away. No luck.

"Oh, I'm sorry," Mom apologized, instinctively grabbing the wheel to propel herself out of the way. Unsuccessful, she sighed, gazing down at the resistant carpet.

"No problem," the man said, kindly waiting as I stood and steered the wheelchair aside. Quickly, he snatched away a magazine.

Mom looked around nervously, clutching her left hand. She studied the flow of people passing by, each secure on healthy legs. Their walking seemed effortless, even to me.

Before long, a tall, pretty blond woman approached and smiled broadly as she greeted Mom. "You must be Agatha Sokol." Leaning down, she took her hand.

Mom smiled back, relaxing. "That's right."

"Well, I'm Ginny, and I'll be your therapist."

They struck up an instant rapport, chatting together as Ginny pushed the wheelchair forward.

The therapy room was spacious, furnished with padded exercise tables and therapy apparatuses all around.

Everything was neat, clean, and maintained a quiet atmosphere.

But Mom was ready for action. "I want to learn how to walk with a quad cane!"

"That's fine," Ginny replied calmly. She eased Mom alongside an exercise table and set the wheelchair brakes. "But how about if we just start with a few exercises first, Agatha?"

"All right." Her enthusiasm tempered, Mom reached up to begin the transfer.

They began with the usual exercises, while I glanced around the room, taking in more of the scene, a motley assortment of human misery. A middle-aged Asian man next to us showed similar signs to Mom's stroke; I was beginning to recognize them. He struggled, walking with his wife's assistance, managing only baby steps as top speed. His right elbow was permanently bent at a right angle. Watching, I prayed for them, somehow encouraged. *At least Mom and I are not alone in our challenge.*

As the man spoke, his speech was slurred, reduced to the mumblings of an infant. I questioned Ginny.

"His stroke was on the right side," she explained. "Your Mom is fortunate she still has her speech."

"That's right," I agreed, though suddenly distracted as Mom pointed to the small, mockup staircase in the middle of the room.

"Can I learn to use the stairs?" She smiled up at Ginny.

"Maybe one of these days." Taking her hand, Ginny negotiated. "First, would you try walking at the railing?"

The wooden bar extended along the full length of a wall. Ginny transferred Mom into the wheelchair and guided her over to it, where we all had a part to play. Mom pushed off from the arm rest and Ginny lifted her to her feet, keeping a hand around her shoulder for balance. I followed behind with the wheelchair, watching as Mom gripped the railing and stepped with her right foot, struggling to initiate the left. Nothing happened. Staring down at her lame foot, she tried again, concentrating, but her fervent mental commands were ignored.

Finally, Ginny reached down and lifted the foot, completing the step. "There, Agatha." She set the foot down. "Now, try the right again."

The same laborious process began. But after only a few minutes and an eight-foot stretch of the railing, Mom's energy drained and she asked to sit. Slumped against the back of the wheelchair, she wiped her brow, sighing, "I never thought I'd have to learn to walk again."

I placed my hand on her shoulder. *I wish she didn't have to go through this. She's already been through so much in her life. Please help her, Blessed Mother.*

Ginny spoke. "Do you have a place to practice walking at home? Like with a railing of some kind?"

"Yes, there's a banister that runs along the hallway upstairs," I replied. "With Dad's help, we can do this same exercise."

The appointment ended. Though Mom was frustrated by her failed walking attempt, she was encouraged to have a wonderful therapist, and proud to have traveled so far from home.

Our next excursion occurred a week later, inspired by a family Kris Kringle tradition. Each year, during Advent, my sister Paula drew names for everyone in the family and informed each of us in a letter who we were to buy a Christmas gift for. When Mom's letter arrived, sealed in a bright green, holiday envelope, I carried it to her, anxious to see her reaction.

"Oh, Paula is such a nut," she said, giggling as she finished reading the humorous verse on the note. She looked up from her pillow and handed it back. "See, I got Anne. But would you mind going shopping and picking out something for me?"

I hinted, aware of another traveling opportunity. "Wouldn't you like to pick it out yourself?"

"No, not really." Disturbed, she looked away.

Why the reluctance? Is it the ride in the car? She didn't mind driving to therapy last week. Still, it seemed best not to push the matter. I slipped the letter back into the envelope. "Let's just see how you feel in the morning."

But when morning arrived, I didn't broach the subject right away. I waited until Mom was washed and dressed, and seated in front of the bathroom mirror where I styled her hair each morning. I picked up the preheated curling iron and worked in the first section of hair, rolling the ends under.

"Don't you think this would be a nice day to go shopping, Mom? It's not raining."

No comment.

The steel hinge creaked as I released the stainless steel wand and worked in the next section of hair.

I continued. "I really think it would be fun. Besides, Anne would love it if you picked out her gift yourself."

Cautiously, Mom reached up and adjusted the drooping left corner of her mouth. "It's so crooked. I'm embarrassed to be seen this way." She turned up a fakey smile, attempting to balance the look.

"Is that the reason you don't want to go shopping, Mom? Really, it doesn't look bad."

She tried again, flashing an even sillier grimace, and asked, "Are you sure?"

I chuckled, fluffing her hair and finishing the effect with hair spray. "You're darling!"

A genuine smile lit her face. "All right, then. Let's go to Nordstrom this morning!"

After breakfast, I bundled her up in an extra-warm sweater and off we went, backing out of the carport like two holiday elves on the loose. Mom's face glowed as I parked at the mall and transferred her from the car. Pushing the wheelchair up the ramped curb, I guided her toward the entry and pulled open the heavy door, propping it open with my hip. Mom extended her hand to help, pressing her palm against the glass. I pushed the wheelchair through, then leapt aside as the door attacked on the back swing. Wham!

We were in, but suddenly time stood still. Two years ago, I had also entered through these same doors with Mom, though brokenhearted and lost. That was the day I left the monastery and she said to me, "Let's go shopping. You need some clothes." Having worn a religious habit for so many years, it was a strange and awkward feeling as we arrived at the mall. I wondered, *Will I fit into regular society again?*

Yes, and with a new purpose. I guided the wheelchair forward, walking slowly. *Two years ago, Mom was also walking—independent, practical, a rock of support.*

I turned the wheelchair into the main corridor and guided her through the teeming crowd. Memories played on. *Even then, physical signs of Mom's weakness were evi-*

dent. For the first time, I saw the effect of the minor stroke she had suffered six years previously. The clip in her step had disappeared and her feet nearly dragged on the ground. I never remarked to her about it at the time, but I remember thinking, Now, I have to slow down for Mom.

I slowed the wheelchair, suddenly faced with the full import of that thought. A frantic mother careened around the corner in pursuit of her two toddler sons. She called out to them as they gleefully raced past us, brushing the side of the wheelchair. Other people also passed by, full of energy and vigor. But Mom, resigned to God's will, moved meekly at her own pace.

"Look at that," I said, viewing a colorful Christmas display before us.

"Oh, it's lovely!" Mom said, pointing to the glittering gold bells and red ribbons hanging above her. "I'm just having so much fun!"

Another woman in a wheelchair glided past and acknowledged us with a nod.

I leaned down to Mom. "See, you're not alone. Now look, here's Nordstrom. Where should I take you?"

"To the jewelry department," she said. "I want to get Anne a necklace."

We made our way toward glass cases near the entry, which gleamed with crystals and pearls. Busy shoppers shuffled through the narrow aisles, but courteously stepped aside to let us pass. Peering through one of the cases now, Mom pointed to an attractive piece.

A clerk noticed and approached. "May I help you?"

Mom handled the whole thing, confident as I

stepped aside to observe. She pointed again. "May I see that pendant, please?"

Bending, the clerk lifted out the necklace of blue and green crystals and handed it to her.

Mom held it high and examined the play of colors through the light. "I think Anne would like this. Don't you, Jenny?"

"Absolutely."

Satisfied, she handed it back to the clerk. "Then I'll take it."

Pleased, she clutched the little shopping bag as we made our way back out into the corridor. Seeing an espresso stand nearby, she pointed, and said, "Let's get something there."

"Sure. And what would you—"

"Hot chocolate!" she answered, anticipating the rest of the question.

I wheeled her to a small, gridiron table and walked toward the counter.

"And don't forget the whipped cream!" she called back.

"I won't." I turned and waved. "Whipped cream coming up."

It crowned the rim, jiggling lightly as I carried the warm cup back to her. Eyes on the goal, she raised the fluffy treat to her lips and sipped slowly.

I sat down, holding my tea. *Mom always loved pumpkin pie, and strawberry shortcake in the summer, topped with a huge dollop of sweetened whipped cream, her favorite.*

I closed my eyes, letting thoughts flow as I rekindled holiday scenes. *She always dressed in flowing hostess gowns on Thanksgiving and Christmas. Even while busy in the kitchen, she looked beautiful as she lifted the pre-chilled stainless steel mixing bowl from the refrigerator and popped the beaters into the portable mixer. She poured a pint of whipped cream into the bowl, sprinkled in sugar—"Just a touch," she taught me, if I was standing near. Then she poured in a few drops of vanilla extract—*

Suddenly, I looked up, vaguely aware that Mom had spoken. "Did you say something?"

She smiled. "I just said I'm sorry to be so slow."

"Not a problem." I picked up her napkin and wiped the creamy mustache from her upper lip. "Take your time."

On the way home we recounted every moment of our adventure, agreeing that a new door of traveling possibilities had opened.

Unable to contain her joy when we bumped through the back doorway at home, Mom blurted out, "I really had a good time, Bill!"

"That's wonderful, sweetie," he said, reaching down to help her with her coat. "How about if we all do the same thing again?"

"That would be wonderful." She pulled her arm from the right sleeve, and asked, "When would be a good time, Jenny?"

"Soon."

Mary's Place

Intertwined in the regular fabric of our daily life, Mary, God's Mother, remained a constant source of hope and strength. Next to the front door in the hallway hung her image as Our Lady of Guadalupe, revealed after winter roses miraculously cascaded from the humble folds of Juan Diego's tilma. In the kitchen, Mary's image was represented in other art pieces, which stood atop cabinets, rested on window sills, or hung from the wall. Each piece was graceful and modest, crafted from far away lands such as Europe, Africa, and Asia. Surrounded by all of these lovely reminders, the thought often occurred that if Mary is everywhere in the world, she was certainly everywhere in our home.

Mary's hand guided my parents from their earliest days together. Even before Mom taught the children the words of the "Hail Mary," she had already tutored Dad in the same prayer during their courtship in the Air Force. The two sat side by side on the Gulf of Mexico sea wall in Biloxi, Mississippi, praying the Rosary. When Dad challenged Mom about Church doctrine, which often involved Mary's place, Mom responded, equal to the task. It wasn't long before Dad took the next step and accepted confirmation into the Catholic Church on the feast of Mary's Assumption, 1945. From that momentous day in August—the definitive end of World War II—until their wedding, 10 days later, my parents never ceased entrusting all of their needs to God through Mary's intercession. Jesus' words "Behold your mother" (John 19:27, Revised New Testament NAB) were manifested as a living person, actively engaged within their marriage.

For Mom, devotion to God's Mother welled from the deepest spring. Following the devastating loss of her own mother, she kept her rosary close at hand, her heart ever listening. Mary, she knew, would guide her forward and keep her close to God.

After the stroke, Mary's image as Our Lady of Mount Carmel hung next to Mom's bed, where she often received Holy Communion by Dad's faithful hand. Seeing Mom's joy at those moments, I was reminded of the angel's mandate to the prophet Elijah: "Get up and eat, else the journey will be too long for you!" (1 Kings 19:7, NAB) Like Mary, the journey was never too lengthy for Mom, nourished as she was by the Bread of Life.

"I've always loved Jesus in the Eucharist," she told me one Sunday morning, smiling. Closing her eyes, she continued her prayer after Communion, immersed in the company of her friend and Savior.

One night, during Mom's initial hospital stay, Mary comforted our trembling hearts. That night I was scheduled to learn bedtime preparations for Mom and stood by her bed waiting for the nurse to come. I glanced at the commode, at Mom, helpless in the wheelchair, then into the bathroom, cheerlessly equipped for the disabled. I battled fear. *Will I be able do this?*

The nurse never came, so Mom finally looked up, and suggested, "Why don't we just go to the chapel. I'd like to pray there."

The idea was inspired. As I guided her from the elevator, then into the quiet, candlelit space, I felt at peace. Looking down at Mom, bundled up in a pink satin bed jacket, with a sheet lightly draped over her legs, I whispered, "Where would you like to go?"

"Over to Our Lady." She pointed to Mary's diminutive statue at the far left corner of the sanctuary. Set slightly behind a tall stand of votive lights, the image shimmered in soft, golden hues as we drew nearer and halted.

Blessed Mother, I prayed, *I don't understand what is happening to Mom, or to me, but I know you'll help us to cope.*

Resting my hand on Mom's shoulder, I drank in the silence, relieved to be far away from the hospital paging system, noisy hallways, and chattering TV's. More than medical help, at the moment we needed God's tender love. Mary had drawn us gently to the fount of mercy.

Our reliance on Mary continued at home, for me, contained in a prayerful nutshell, *I'm all yours,* and for Mom through her favorite devotion, the Rosary. Meditation upon the fifteen mysteries accompanied everything she did.

One morning, as I entered her room to "Do the Exercises" as the time came to be known, as usual I found her praying along with her group Rosary tape.

"Are you ready to do the exercises?" I asked.

"What?" Clutching the beads, she reached to shut off the tiny cassette machine lying on her tummy. She glanced up. "Wait." The black wooden beads rattled against the machine as she engaged the off switch. More rattling as the beads caught in the cord and she fumbled to pull the mini headphone away from her right ear. Successful, she said, "Say that again."

"Are you ready to do the exercises now?"

"Almost. Just let me finish the Sorrowfuls first."

She released the headphone, which snapped neatly back to her ear. Without looking down, she switched on the recorder and continued to meditate. Silently, she lipped the Hail Marys.

Meanwhile, seeing her left hand caught under the tape machine, I reached and lifted it away. Mom, smiling, nodded, used to these frequent limb adjustments. Kneeling, I lifted the bedspread fringe from the floor and checked under the bed. As suspected, the Chap Stick had fallen again, knocked from the bed table during a foiled, one-handed effort by Mom to smooth it on during the night.

The tape machine clicked off. Standing, I looked at Mom.

"Okay, I'm ready," she said, pulling the headphones off. "Let's go."

I set the tape machine on the dresser, transferred her into the wheelchair, and guided her into Dad's room where we always did the exercises. Proficient with transfers, Mom reached smoothly for her dangling left arm and held it as I let her down onto the bed. Already, her right foot, covered with a white sock, was going.

"One . . . two . . . three . . ." she counted, rhythmically bending the ankle up and down, proud to "show off" her working muscles. She looked sideways, searching my face for approval.

"Very good."

Reaching "ten," she began to work the left foot,

though a much more challenging process. "How's that?" She glanced at her feet, peering through the bottom of her large, wire-rimmed bifocals. "Is it any better?"

"Pretty good."

But we both knew the difficult truth. The left muscles were poor and showed no sign of improvement. I bent down and gently leaned my palm into the ball of her foot, completing the full range of upward motion. We counted the remaining lifts together. "Eight . . . nine . . . ten."

"Let's do this one now," she said, trying to pull both knees up.

But the left one lagged. I reached under the knee and guided it the rest of the way. With both knees in position, Mom began to do pelvis rolls from side to side.

But haven't we done all of this a thousand times before? Feeling monotony set in, I prayed for patience, and reached for Mom's left knee. I nudged the unresponsive hip over the rest of the way.

"Do you think it's getting any better?" she asked.

I hesitated, unsure of how to respond. *What kind of hope can I offer? Any?*

"No," I finally replied. "But it's not any worse. You're doing the best you can."

I stood and stepped around to the foot of the bed, waiting as Mom lifted her good knee to a right angle in the air. Ten times she pushed into the palm of my hand. I resisted the motion, working the muscles. The right leg was strong, but not the left.

"Whew!" she said, finally stopping as she drew the back of her hand to her forehead. "That's really hard work."

"It is," I agreed, letting her leg down and folding

my arms. "How about resting? I think it would be a good idea."

I sat down at the foot of the bed and looked at her. For some reason, the session had seemed particularly tedious. Feeling the same way, Mom looked over at the small, wooden statue of Mary on the dresser, and sighed softly. Thinking she was praying for courage, or perhaps for a miracle, I was surprised when she suddenly laughed and stammered out the next words.

"My real problem is. . . . I hate to exercise!"

"I noticed," I said, grateful for the lighthearted change of pace.

"The one thing I always loved to do, though," she continued, "was to play tennis."

Relaxing, she crossed her right ankle over her left and described the teenage memory with her brother Leo.

"We used to play for hours," she said. "We'd get up at the crack of dawn and walk down the road to a private club. We snuck under the fence and played for about an hour and a half, then left before anyone discovered us. Afterward, we went out and ate ice cream for breakfast!"

More laughter.

"You and Dad used to play tennis, too, didn't you?"

"Yes," Mom replied, growing quieter as a tinge of longing entered her voice. "We did quite a bit of that when we were young." She paused, looking toward the window. "Gosh, when I think of how I used to be able to run around like that."

I waited, wishing I could restore her walking. But reality dictated otherwise. *No use dwelling on If Only's.*

I stood. "How about finishing the exercises now?"

"Fine," she said, uncrossing her ankles and slipping

her right hand beneath her head on the pillow. She lifted her right leg slightly from the mattress and extended it out to the side, working the inner thigh muscles. The left leg refused to budge, so I lifted it and completed the motion.

"It's pretty bad, isn't it?" Mom said.

"Yes. But it's still important to move. Any kind of exercise will help maintain your muscle tone and stamina."

Weeks of therapy wore on without any improvement. Some days were better than others. But increasingly, I looked to Mary, praying for grace. *Please help us to accept reality. Mom isn't getting any better. Show us the way.*

On a significant day—February 11, the feast of Our Lady of Lourdes—Mom and I arrived at the outpatient therapy appointment in the hospital. The day had been especially anticipated, because Ginny promised Mom to fulfill her ongoing dream and allow her to walk alone with a quad cane. Adding to the drama, Ginny promised Mom that she could walk in the room's open floor space. No railing! Mom could hardly wait.

She glowed as Ginny wheeled her away from the exercise table, then out into the middle of the floor. All around, heads turned; the "regulars" in the room were not about to miss Agatha's big moment. Several people moved in closer to watch.

"Here we go," Ginny said, tugging on the transfer belt.

Lips pursed, eyes focused on her legs, Mom pushed off from the arm rest as Ginny pulled her to her feet. Taking hold of the aluminum quad cane handle, Mom looked down at her feet, and pronounced, "See, Jenny! I'm going to walk!"

Rarely had I witnessed such excitement in her. Standing slightly behind, I observed as Ginny coached, keeping an arm around Mom's shoulder. Secure, Mom stepped forward with her right foot, then independently lifted her left foot for the first time.

"Good, Agatha! Great!" everyone exclaimed, applauding as Mom set her foot down on the floor again.

"Yes, good, Mom," I said, though reserved. How could I be excited when she was already sitting again, her energy drained? *Will it ever return?*

"Wasn't that good, Jenny?" she asked, beaming as she looked up from the wheelchair.

"Yes, you did really well, Mom."

More of her fans congratulated her as I bent down, and asked, "Do you think you can make it to Mass now?"

"Oh, yes," she replied, confidently tapping the arm rest. "I almost forgot. Right away."

The special liturgy, offered on Mary's feast for the sick, was about to begin in the hospital chapel. We excused ourselves, made our way to the upper floor, and entered the sacred space. I wheeled Mom alongside a front pew and stepped inside, kneeling to pray. But I struggled inwardly. While Mom was here to celebrate her one magnificent step, I was not. Realizing her inability to even boost herself from a chair, how could I realistically hope that she would walk again? Was I the only skeptic? The stubborn pessimist? At that moment, I could only pray in one way. *Whatever Mom's future holds, help her, Blessed Mother. Obtain for us healing grace, however we need it.*

Or, as Mom always said in life's darkest moments: "Whatever God wants."

Sadly, she never repeated her independent walking

again. No matter how great her desire, or the laborious effort that she poured into it, her left leg never responded. The day finally arrived, almost exactly a year to the date of her celebrated one step, when I felt the need to talk privately with Ginny. While Mom rested after the therapy session, the two of us stepped aside into Ginny's office and spoke frankly.

"It seems to me," I began, relieved to finally unburden my mind, "that we're just spinning our wheels. Mom isn't making any progress. Am I right?"

Ginny sighed. "I'm afraid not. Your mother will never regain the use of her arm, or her leg. I'm sorry."

"So, is there any point in coming here again?"

"No, probably not. But you should keep on doing the exercises at home. That will do Agatha some good."

Obviously, we had both been thinking the same thing for a long time, holding out hope for improvement. Still, I wondered about Mom and her reaction. *Will she spiral into a depression?*

She looked toward me sweetly as Ginny and I approached. She continued to gaze steadily as we relayed the results of our conversation. Half expecting a quarrel, I was relieved when nothing of the sort happened.

"I understand," Mom said simply, resigned to the truth. Then, looking at Ginny, she said, "Thank you for your help. You've done a very good job. I'll always pray for you."

That was all. Exchanging embraces with our wonderful friend, we returned to the car and never regretted our time with her.

Later that evening, as I sat on the kitchen couch, thoughts about Mom whirled through my head. Though certain about our decision to end outpatient therapy, the moment presented yet another opportunity to let go and accept Mom's limited future. *Help her to cope.*

Just then, from down the hallway in her room, I heard my parents laughing together.

As always, able to find the bright side in every trial.

In the next minute, I heard Dad intone the familiar invocation: "In the name of the Father, and of the Son, and of the Holy Spirit . . ."

Recognizing they had started the Rosary, I joined in. *Holy Mary, Mother of God.*

Watery Woes

The day had started out as usual. I washed and dressed Mom, fed her breakfast, and changed the bed linens. Calmly, I carried out each chore without interruption. But an hour later, everything changed as my physical and emotional gears were suddenly thrust into reverse and I sank to my knees, head buried under the laundry room sink, desperately trying to stop a stream of hot water blasting from a burst pipe. I struggled to shut off the valve, thwarted by the water's scalding temperature. Repeatedly, I reached, then pulled my arm back again. Finally, thinking my efforts were for nothing, I stood and wiped my wet face, praying, *Now, what do I do?*

At that moment, I heard the sound of heavy feet bound through the door behind me. Reeling around, I stared in disbelief at a man who stood, staring back. I gasped. "Who are YOU?"

Without responding, the unknown visitor, dressed in jeans, a flannel work shirt, and what looked like a painter's hat, motioned for me to step aside. Dropping to his knees, he grabbed a crumpled, wet towel lying on the floor and used it to shield his hands and face. A few swift cranks on the valve and the water stopped.

Praise God!

Standing, the man faced me, professional as a soldier who had just completed a mission. He answered my previous question. "I'm a plumber. Your sister came and got me."

"You mean Anne?" I paused, perplexed. "But she's been here all morning. Where did she find you?"

"I guess she noticed my business truck parked at the neighbor's house when she drove in. When you called upstairs for help, she ran next door and got me. She's with your mother now."

"Thank you," I said, amazed at the providential turn of events. "You certainly saved the day."

From up in the kitchen, Mom called down the stairs. "Is everything all right, Jenny?"

"Almost." I stared at the open cupboard, the severed pipe, and the leftover puddle at my feet. *Just another water adventure.*

"Will that be all, then?" the plumber asked.

"Yes, thank you. Now, what do we owe you?"

"Nothing," he said, turning as he adjusted his cap, then climbed back up the stairs.

Hearing him leave through the back door, I called back up to Mom. "It's just like Tacoma. Remember?"

"Tacoma" was a never-to-be-forgotten episode, named for a city south of Seattle. Shortly after I began taking care of Mom, I was called to play an orchestra job there, which involved a fair driving distance, about 50 miles from home. Under the circumstances, the logistics presented a sizable feat, but Mom insisted that I go. As far as she was concerned, I needed to keep up a normal life by getting out to play my violin. But "normal" to me meant to " . . . seek first the kingdom of God. " (Matthew 6:33, Revised New Testament NAB) Since Mom was "first" on my list in the kingdom, I considered everything else as secondary. Still, after more thought, I decided to give it a try and weigh the results.

The idea was simple. Before leaving for the job, I would get Mom up and fed, then back into bed. By the time I returned home at noon, I would help her with the commode. In the meantime, Dad would keep watch. And that's how it worked out—barely.

The job's one and only rehearsal fell on a Saturday morning. Just after sunrise, I entered Mom's room and found her awake, ready to carry out our little plan. We tried to be especially quiet, so as not to waken Dad. Moving swiftly, I washed Mom, transferred her onto the commode, then crept across the hallway into the bathroom, carrying the commode bucket. No matter what, I had to move quickly.

Suddenly, everything backfired. As I flushed the toilet, something in the mechanism snapped, and water began to gush from both the tank and the bowl. Before I knew it, we were into a deluge.

"Oh no!" I called out. "The toilet's broken. There's water going everywhere!"

"Oh, my God," Mom returned, her voice weak.

I panicked. Knowing she was half dressed and helpless on the commode, what could I do? *Nothing!* I forged ahead.

Pulling open the cupboard door below the sink, I pulled out an armful of old bath towels. Just then, Dad, dressed in pajamas, stumbled sleepily through the doorway. His wavy, silver hair was a moppy mess.

"What's going on?" he asked.

"It's the toilet," I answered, shoving several towels into his arms.

Quickly, he sized up the situation and unfurled the first one, tossing it to the wet floor. Squirming past him, I ran to check on Mom, now listing precariously left on the commode. Her bare back faced me from the doorway. "Are you okay?"

"Yes, fine," she replied softly, holding her left arm in her lap. "I wish I could help."

Satisfied she could bear up a minute longer, I whirled around and eyed the rivulet fast paving a pathway for her door. The toilet churned, hissing menacingly in the background. I stooped, damming up Mom's doorway with towels, then skidded past Dad in the bathroom to fix the toilet. I lifted the tank lid away and set it on the floor. Clank! Thrusting my arm into the frigid water, I tinkered with each part, having no idea what I was looking for. Finally, pulling up on a stick—the one with the floating black ball attached to it—the flow of water ceased. Not to risk a recap, I reached down and lifted the toilet brush, propped against the wall. I jammed the handle underneath the stick and secured it in place. Releasing my right-handed hold, I called out, "The water stopped!"

"Thank God," Mom weakly returned.

I sloshed back to her side and found her remarkably tranquil, a seasoned expert in time of trial. *If only I could be so composed.*

Completing the hastier than usual dressing, I wheeled her into the kitchen, served breakfast, then ran downstairs to get a mop from the laundry room closet. *This will only take a minute. Enough time to help Dad with the cleanup, then leave for Tacoma.*

But just as I ran through the laundry room door and flicked on the light, there it was—*More water!*—leaked from the bathroom above. The last drips plopped pathetically from the ceiling light fixture, adding to the puddle on the floor. I glanced at the clock. *No time.* But with little choice, I grabbed the mop and began to swab. By the time things were dry, only minutes remained to jump in the shower, dress, and get Mom back into bed. Before leaving, I prayed, *Just get me there on time.*

I backed out of the carport and headed for the freeway. Miraculously, I made it to Tacoma on time. But as I took my seat in the small orchestra, surrounded by new faces and circumstances, I felt like a foreigner in a strange land. Concerns at home pressed in. *How are Mom and Dad? Was it right to accept this job? Perhaps these gigs are too much right now . . . Dad will soon learn the transfers, but maybe Mom needs me closer.* I struggled to suppress my inner turmoil as the conductor signaled and I lifted my bow. The rest of the rehearsal was pure effort.

Back at home and well into the evening, things were relatively back to normal. But not without significant consequence beforehand. Mom had not done well while I was away, so the two of us were holding an impromptu discernment session in her room.

"I don't think I should play any more gigs," I said, seated cross-legged on the chest at the foot of her bed.

"Then I'll be taking you away from your fun, too," she said.

"Well, I won't be having any fun if you're miserable at home."

A long pause followed before she responded. "Well, just see what you think."

The next evening brought the answer. Immediately following the concert in Tacoma, I drove home, though nagged by a buzzing, uneasy feeling inside. *Is Mom in trouble?*

She called out as soon as I stepped through the back door. "Jenny, please come!"

Nearly dropping my violin case, I rushed to her room and stood by her side. There, with ponytail resting atop the pillow, Mom was flustered and shaken, only the light from the hallway illuminating the surroundings.

"What's wrong?" I asked, kicking off my black high-heels and fumbling to remove my coat. I backed up and tossed it over the wheelchair behind me, my eyes fixed on Mom.

"Oh, I don't know," she said, randomly gesticulating with her hand. "I'm just all upset. I'm so glad you're home."

I shifted into nursing mode and checked her blood pressure. Sure enough, it was elevated. But she had already taken her medication that day, so I walked around to the right side of the bed and laid down beside her. *Perhaps this is the best medicine right now. She's traumatized like a child in the night.* "It's okay, Tiny Person," I said, taking her hand.

The feel of her soft, slender fingers rested like a warm memory within my own. How often in my childhood had she comforted me with her mother's touch?

"I thought you would never come home again," she said, flushed with emotion.

"I won't leave you," I promised. "And I'm not going to play anymore jobs."

"Are you sure?"

"Yes, at least for now. You need me. This is where I belong."

At peace, I felt the urge to offer my mother the same gift. Quietly, I recounted a childhood memory for her. "There was a huge storm one night," I began. "I was only six, but I remember it like it happened yesterday."

Awake in bed, I was terrified by the sound of wind whipping in harrowing whistles through our two gigantic poplar trees, located just outside my window. Any second, I thought, the trees would crash onto the house. Too afraid to bear the suspense any longer, I rose from my bed and knocked on my parents' bedroom door.

"What is it?" Mom asked, standing in the unlit doorway.

"I'm scared," I whispered, looking up. "I think the trees are going to fall on the house."

She chuckled, reassuring me, "The trees are very strong. I don't think they will fall on the house."

Embracing me, she sent me back to bed, my fear relieved.

"Do you remember that?" I asked her, still holding her hand.

"No," she replied. "But I'm feeling better."

The day's turbulence had subsided, but not the water problems. For some reason they kept trickling in all along the way of our journey. As Mom and I waded in and out of our soggy perils, the psalmist's cry often came to mind: "Save me, O God, for the waters have risen to my neck!" (Psalm 69:1, NEB)

One afternoon, finding ourselves nearly up to our scruffs in a swimming pool, our watery episodes reached a new high. The pool idea had seeped into the scheme of things early on, the recommendation of a therapist.

"Swimming therapy may help you, Agatha," she told her. "Why don't you give it a try?"

That was enough to instill a permanent bug in Mom's ear, never to leave until her toes were at last dipped into the public pool's warm water. As tenacious as her enthusiasm, though, was my aversion. Having endured an endless litany of therapeutic suggestions after outpatient therapy ended, I was worn out by false hopes and concomitant disappointments. Mom's adamant pleas to "At least try, Jenny," finally won out, and we again headed to the mall, this time in search of a bathing suit.

For sure, the swimsuit shop was no handicapped haven as we strolled through the neon-lit entrance and discovered a small, tightly packed space of beachwear glamour. We narrowly made our way past short racks of colorful bikinis and sexy sarongs.

"What do you think?" I teased, holding up a tiger-striped design.

"Not exactly," Mom replied, grinning. "But how about one of those?"

She pointed to the more conservative rack along the wall. Before long, we made two selections—blue ones—and crammed ourselves into a tiny fitting room, huffing and puffing our way through the inescapable realities of spacial limitations.

"Sorry about this." Pinned against the mirror, I faced Mom and struggled to pull her left arm from the shirt sleeve. My right elbow banged against the wall.

I stooped, squeezed into the corner, and removed her shoes; the rug was filthy. Wary, my mind projected into the future. *What will the pool be like? Will the facilities be clean?* I stood and wiped my overheated brow. *The therapist told us that the therapy classes take place in between regular swimming classes. Will the dressing rooms accommodate the disabled? I bet not.*

The whole idea loomed more and more like an inevitable disaster. But quiet attempts at reason only fell on deaf ears. In Mom's estimation, anything was possible.

"I don't mind, Jenny," she kept telling me, determined.

I struggled to lift her and adjust the swimsuit. *How can she be so sure?* Again, my elbow met the wall.

"I have to do this," Mom continued. She lifted her right arm as I adjusted the shoulder strap. "I'll never know until I try."

I climbed over the wheelchair's left armrest and stepped out of the way. Helping Mom to stand, I kept a firm hold around her shoulders.

She viewed herself in the mirror. "Let's get this one."

There was no turning back. Guiding her back to the car, we headed for home, committed to the end.

But to the end, nothing followed that proverbial path of roses. When the scheduled day for the therapy class arrived, so did a wind and rain storm, portending with more certainty the shape of things to come.

"Perfect," I mused dryly, staring out of Mom's bedroom window at the gathered gloom and pelting precipitation. Though an early spring afternoon, the effect appeared more like an early winter evening. "Are you sure you don't want to put this off until another day, Mom?" I turned and faced her, visualizing the whole thing: traffic jams, blustery car transfers, Mom getting soaked in the wheelchair.

"No, let's go," she said, resolved as she looked up from her pillow. "And I want to wear pantyhose."

"Pantyhose!"

Mom hadn't worn full-length hose since the stroke; it was too hard to pull them on and off. *Besides, she only wears slacks now. Why pantyhose?*

I tried to convince her otherwise, but she insisted. "I'll feel much better if my legs are covered."

I lifted a pair from her former dresser and returned to her room, where she was waiting in the wheelchair. Sweating, I struggled to inch the extra-support spandex up her yet full-figured body. While she balanced against me, I fought to keep both of us upright before completing the task, letting her down, and collapsing into a heap on the bed.

"Do you realize we'll have to repeat this at the pool, Mom?"

She did.

The small equipment bag rested in her lap as I pushed the wheelchair down the hallway. We bumpety-bumped through the back doorway and were immediately met by a gust from the gale. I watched as sheets of rain pummelled the driveway. *Mother of God, help us.*

I transferred Mom into the car, climbed into the driver's seat, and started the engine. Ready or not, we were on our way.

The pool was located about 30 minutes from home. As thunder and lightning increased, so did my apprehension. Things were not looking good, at least from my perspective. I rounded the final corner and suspiciously eyed the cement building. "This is the place. Let's hope the handicapped parking spaces are close to the entrance."

Not so. The entrance was invisible from the busy thoroughfare, and the only apparent parking lot was set at the far end of the block. Pulling in, I backed into the sole handicapped space, which followed up a slight incline, and turned off the engine.

What could have been a simple stroll to the entrance, became a mountainous trek. Through the driving wind, I dug the wheelchair from the trunk and planted it beside the muddy embankment. Lunging, I grabbed it as it began to roll away, watching as muck splattered in between the wheel spokes.

I spun the wheelchair around and pushed it alongside Mom's car door, shouting orders as we carried out the tilted transfer. Even with the gale threatening to carry away Mom's little umbrella, she never complained, and held onto it tightly as she sat down in the wet seat.

I guided her forward, hoping to find the building entrance nearby. *But where?* I turned onto the sidewalk and stopped, scanning the scene. *No door in sight.* The storm and traffic noise only added to my confusion, and I shouted to anyone in heaven or on earth willing to listen, "Where's the front door of this place, anyway?"

I looked to the right. The building's unusual pyramid-like structure had grassy, sloped sides and paved pathways, which led up to a flat-topped sort of mesa. *The entrance?*

Lacking any clue, I took the chance of finding it and began to climb. It was hard going as I fought gravity and the storm, pushing Mom in her wheelchair up the steep incline. "We're almost there!" I shouted, leaning more heavily into the wheelchair handles. "Don't worry, Mom."

But just as we crested the top, thinking the end was in sight, I heard her plaintive cry. "I don't have my footrest on!" At the same moment, the umbrella blew inside out. Thwack!

"Jesus, save us!" I yelled, looking heavenward as I burst into laughter. Overcome by the sight of our two windblown figures, I could only think of the famous storm-at-sea episode from the Gospel. Though on land, Jesus, I knew, was in "the boat." But he would have to forgive my unfortunate oversight about the footrest. Left in the car, there was no time to retrieve it.

"Just cross your left ankle under your right!" I called down to Mom. "And try to keep your heels off the ground!"

But she hardly heard me. Unshielded from the elements, she too was laughing, tussling the umbrella as rain soaked through her clothes.

"God . . . is my shield," I said, as the psalmist's words came to mind (Psalm 7:10, NEB). I removed my jacket and draped it over Mom's head. *Now what do we do?*

With no entrance in sight, I guided the wheelchair back down the hill. Gravity figured in all the more as I leaned back, struggling to control my heavy load.

"Are your feet up?" I yelled.

"I'm trying!" Mom called back.

Reaching the sidewalk, I guided the wheelchair down to the far end the block and peered to the right. *The entrance!* Carved like a cave into the side of the building, it finally came into view.

I pushed Mom through the automatic doors and

stopped, savoring the silence. "Are you all right?" I lifted the coat from her head as she uncrossed her feet.

"Yes, fine, but tired. That's a lot of work without a footrest."

We made our way to the dressing room and sought privacy, but none was available. No such thing as even a curtain. My own needs were not a problem, but Mom was embarrassed and felt like a misfit among the other women, all young, strong, and able-bodied. Chatting, they stood near lockers, or sat on wooden benches, which filled the room's middle area.

The cement walls and floor amplified their high-pitched voices, so Mom and I settled at a bench furthest from the hub. We spoke in undertones, ignoring their curious stares as I lifted Mom up and down to remove her outer garments.

"Almost done," I said, fastening her hair up into a large clip and fitting the bathing cap over her head. It snapped into place. "Like the snap in this air." I shivered, seized with cold. I scrambled to change my own clothes, then stooped, stuffing everything back into the equipment bag. I zipped it closed and attempted to conceal it beneath the bench.

"I'll pray nobody walks off with it," Mom said.

The smell of chlorine hung thickly in the warm, humid air as I wheeled her out to the pool area. A blue-and-white striped rope floated in the shallow end, marking the class location. I met the eyes of several other attendees who were standing nearby, but no one offered a welcoming word. *Are they newcomers as well?* I smiled, turning to the man next to me and decided to initiate the effort. "Hello."

No reply.

Right. Every man for himself. I backed Mom against the wall and waited in silence.

Soon, a young woman, the instructor, appeared from the locker room and confidently strode past. She wore a bathing suit, a yellow baseball cap, and poised a whistle between her lips. As she stopped next to the yellow chair lift in the corner of the pool, several people in wheelchairs swarmed to her side like a school of fish. I guided Mom to the end of the line and watched as the chair lift hummed into action. One by one, down they went, mostly elderly "swimmers."

Pushing Mom alongside the chair lift, I spoke to the instructor. "We're new here. I wonder if you could tell us—"

But she cut me off, rattling off directions to Mom. Frustrated, I gave up and stepped in front of the wheelchair. *Just follow the crowd.* I transferred Mom into the chair lift, secured the seat buckle, then climbed down into the pool. Mom, fearless, smiled as the chair lift lowered her into the water.

"I'm here," she sighed, pleased by the weightless feel of her body as I helped her to her feet.

"Kind of like Chevy Chase, isn't it?" I led her forward, lightly holding onto the transfer belt.

"Yes," she said, reminded of our former family vacation spot. She looked down, studying her limbs, which painted illusory figures beneath the water's blue ripples. "I taught you to swim at Chevy Chase, remember?"

"Yes. How could I ever forget?" I pictured Mom again as she gently guided my first paddles. I was terrified, but she was a much braver student now than I was then.

"Just take it slowly," I said, patting her shoulder. "Let's stop here."

We stood at the back of the group, watching as the instructor waded vigorously past to the front. Facing us, she gave a loud blast on the whistle and delivered her terse opener. "First, the right leg! Ready?"

The veterans set in, swinging their legs in a memorized pattern. I described the motion to Mom, but she struggled to imitate it.

I raised my hand, signaling for the instructor. "Could you show my mother, please? She's never been here before."

She darted a glance, and called out, "Just do the best you can and work with her at her own pace. Most of these people have been coming for a long time."

Annoyed, I whispered, "I don't think we fit in here."

"I guess she's got better things to do," Mom said, half teasing as she began to improvise, moving her legs like a venerable ballerina in slow motion. The skirt of her bathing suit spread like a tutu beneath the water. I supported her from under the arms, watching the "dance." *At least she can enjoy a few minutes in her carefree, artistic world.*

But as the class pace quickened, so did the difficulty of the required movements. That meant less activity and more pauses in between for Mom.

"I think I'd better stop now," she finally said, content to stand still. Goose bumps quickly formed across her shoulders.

She'll freeze when we get out of the pool. Dressing her quickly will be difficult. What about the toilet? Should I take

*her to use the bathroom immediately after we get out of the
pool, or should I wait until she's dressed? Maybe I should wait
until she's home. I can't put her through too much . . . Oh, God,
this is too much!* As never before, I felt my caregiving limits
and knew I could never do this again.

Class ended and I guided Mom back to the chair
lift where we waited in line. When our turn finally came,
I helped Mom into the seat, then climbed from the pool.
Our teeth chattered in unison as we went through the
slippery transfer and she slid down into the wheelchair.

"Here." I lifted the towel from my shoulder and
wrapped it around her.

She pulled it tightly together, pressing it high
around her neck. "Oh, it's cold!"

In the dressing room, everything was wet: our bod-
ies, the furniture, clothes, the cold cement floor.

"I have to get you warm before anything else," I told
Mom. "Here, stand up. Let's get these wet things off."

But as I lifted her from the wheelchair, she lost
control and urinated through her bathing suit onto the
floor. I held her closer as my eyes filled with tears. *This is
the last straw.*

I dressed her quickly, sidestepping the puddle. The
room's stillness set in and I looked around. *Is there anyone
here to help? At least to locate a cleaning detergent to wash the
floor?* But everyone had left and we were all alone. I knelt,
picking up one of our wet towels and performed the inad-
equate cleaning job. I felt like a failure. "Probably anyone
else in the world would be better at this than I."

"Don't feel badly," Mom said, leaning over and
stroking my head.

I stuffed the soiled towel into the equipment bag.

"You didn't know this would happen."

As some measure of relief, the storm had died down by the time we drove home. But I was still upset and needed to communicate my distress to Mom. "I can't do this again," I told her. "It's too much for me."

"But I really enjoyed being in the pool! I think it will help."

"I know you liked the water. But getting you here . . . the weather . . . the pantyhose . . . the lousy dressing room arrangement . . . not being able to keep up with the class pace . . . I feel crazy even thinking that we might have to do this again."

The conversation turned into a full-fledged argument, the biggest we would ever have. It was doubly hard, because I didn't want to hurt Mom who had so little in her life. *Am I just being selfish?*

Time and prayer eventually "calmed the sea" for both of us, and it didn't take long. That evening, after dinner, I checked on Mom. She was watching an old, black-and-white movie on the portable TV in her room and hit the mute button on the remote control as I approached.

She looked up and spoke before I could get a word out. "I don't need to go to the pool anymore, Little One. I know it's too much for you."

Not to dwell on the matter, I thanked her simply, then added, "But I promise I'll keep helping you with exercises at home. Even without professional therapy, they're important to do."

"I know," she said, smiling. Reaching for her cup, she handed it to me. "Could you fill it with fresh water, please?"

"Of course."

The Room

"Wait, Jenny. My trees."

"Your trees?" I asked, turning. "What are you talking about?"

Mom's room was dark, lit only by the hallway light. After checking on her for the final time that night, I had started to leave, when she pointed to the drapery, and explained, "I can't see my trees. Could you pull it open a little more, please?"

Though often overlooked by me, I now noted the patch of evergreens just outside the window, modestly silhouetted against the night sky. Drawing the drapery open a few more inches, I again realized how limited Mom's world had become. After three years of lying in bed, the small poetic comfort provided by "her trees" was precious.

"Thank you," she said, as I completed the task and walked toward her. "That's better."

I kissed her on the forehead and adjusted her left arm under the covers. Meanwhile, her right hand began the pat-and-feel search for her rosary, again hidden among the blanket folds. We laughed; how many times had we been through this before?

"Could you help me?" she asked, enjoying the moment.

Lifting the covers, I located the rosary, mysteriously hidden under her right shoulder, and handed it to her. Leaving, I turned at the door with a final "goodnight" and stood still to watch as she silently prayed. Fingering the beads, her eyes were fixed on the window. She was the picture of peace.

The ivory drapes were among the few furnishings in Mom's room. Hanging to the floor along the full width of the wall at the foot of her bed, they were never parted. Otherwise, bright daylight streamed in, blinding Mom whose only view was straight into the sky. Through her "peek hole" in the drapes, she stayed in touch with a little piece of nature, comforted by the beauty. She grew accustomed to every movement of the tiny house sparrows, which flitted in and out of the house eaves during nesting season. She often remarked about certain ones as if they were friends, pointing toward the left side of the window.

"That little guy has been hauling in straw all day long."

Another bird flew in and perched on the same eave.

"Isn't that one cute? I think it's the scout."

Having lived in a cloister, I understood the dynamics of a small living space. One's world, contained within an exceptionally compact area, either becomes highly valued or impossibly annoying, depending upon each person. In Mom's case, she loved the quiet, personal atmosphere of her home, as opposed to a nursing home. But still, it was the little things that she stared at all day in her room——or rather, which stared back at her——that sometimes got the upper hand and grated on her nerves.

"Would you straighten that pleat?" she asked one

evening, pointing to the top section of the drapery immediately in front of her.

I had just entered the room and stopped, following her fingertip with my gaze toward the mark.

"There are lots of pleats," I said, focusing more intently as I studied the cotton brocade's obscure, paisley pattern. "They all look the same to me."

"No," she said, gesturing more emphatically. "See, the one overlapping that one a little? It's been driving me crazy for days. Please, just do what I say. Climb up there and I'll show you."

I pulled the desk chair over and stepped onto it, pointing for clarification. "This one?"

"No," she said, dropping the back of her hand to her forehead. "One more over."

I had it. Giving the fabric a miniscule tug downward, the neighboring pleats evened out.

"Oh, thank you!" Mom sighed, clasping her hand to her heart, as if an enormous weight had been lifted.

I climbed down and slid the chair back into place under the desk.

"You don't know what it's like to look at the same things day after day," Mom said, picking up her booklet to continue her prayers.

But I did know, and prayed for her, realizing all too well the challenges of confinement.

"You're really living the life of a contemplative, you know," I said, dragging the black canister vacuum cleaner behind me as I walked through her doorway one morning—the time had come for my weekly cleaning chore. "You're like Mary listening to Jesus, and I'm 'Martha,

Martha . . . anxious and upset about many things'" (Luke 10:41, NAB).

We laughed.

"Do you mind if I run the vacuum now? This will only take a few minutes."

"No, that's fine," Mom said, setting her rosary and tape machine aside on the bed table. She pondered my previous remark. "I guess I do pray a lot."

I parted the drapery in the middle and placed my foot over the power switch on the vacuum cleaner. Turning it on, I worked the dusting attachment across the high window sill, then vacuumed the hinged screen attached to a separate window at the far right. Bird feathers and straw had collected during the flurry of warm weather activity. Nestlings, hidden just out of sight in the eaves, reacted in a chorus of shrill cheeps, protesting the sonic invasion.

"They make a mess, don't they?" Mom commented, watching the distraction with amusement.

A fresh collection of molted gray-and-white feathers floated past the window.

I closed the drapes and attached the power head to the vacuum. Noisily it surged forward over the narrow space between the bed table and wall, clacking as fallen Tylenol pills were swept inside. Backing around the foot of the bed, I misjudged the tight corner and dove to free the bedspread tassels, which were instantly sucked in and snared around the roller. "Darn it! Did it again." I cut the motor and upended the power head, freeing the elongated strings.

Mom chuckled. "No great loss. That bedspread is as old as you kids."

"Like all of the furniture in here," I said, eyeing the

blond-wood dresser, once part of my childhood bedroom furnishings.

I followed to the matching desk at the left and studied the gracefully fluted ceramic lamp, formerly a living room feature. The stem, painted with a sprig of dogwood, supported a delicate peach-colored lamp shade and added elegance to the otherwise plain room.

I pulled the vacuum cleaner past the wheelchair and commode, both parked in front of the desk, and aimed the power head toward the worn section of carpeting alongside Mom's bed.

"It's practically threadbare," I said, raising my voice as I stepped on the power switch again. "But it will have to do. I've shampooed it so many times."

I finished the five-foot section of carpeting between the bed and closet, pulled the cord from the hallway outlet, and rewound the cord.

"Could you please hand me one of my scripture tapes now?" Mom asked, pointing to the dresser.

I reached over the wheelchair. "Is Mother Katherine Sullivan all right?" I held up one of the scripture scholar's lecture tapes.

"Yes, fine," Mom said. "I get so much out of her ideas."

I handed her the cassette machine, watching as she positioned the headphones around her ears. Tuned into the spiritual talk, she soon tuned me out, eyes closed, imbibing spiritual nourishment according to St. John of the Cross, the Carmelite mystic:

In the inner wine cellar
I drank of my Beloved . . .
(from *The Spiritual Canticle,* St. John of the Cross)

After the stroke, Mom's inner life intensified. Prayer and the offering of her sufferings, in union with those of Jesus, comprised her entire purpose and imbued her helplessness with the overriding power of God's redemptive love. But not without God's merciful preparation beforehand. Alike to Jesus' Transfiguration on Mount Tabor before his imminent Passion and Death, Mom experienced her own "mountaintop," and shared the experience one morning as we spoke.

"For five years you haven't had privacy in the bathroom," I said, helping her off the commode. "I have to do everything for you, but you never mind. How can you be so patient?"

Without hesitating, she explained. "About a week before the stroke, I was standing in front of the refrigerator, when suddenly I was enveloped by an overwhelming aroma of incense. I had never experienced anything like that, so I knelt down and thanked God. I felt God so close to me, and how much I was loved. I think it must have lasted a minute or so. When I stood up again, I just kept on with whatever I was doing; I didn't know what else to do. But I never forgot about it, and kept thanking God for the next several days. Then the stroke came . . ."

Like the experience she described, her face was lit with joy.

"It sounds like an anointing," I said.

"Yes, maybe that's what you'd call it. But whatever it was, it helped me so much to think of it right after the stroke. I knew that God loved me, and wanted me to accept everything and to offer it with love."

"God is very close to you," I said, kissing her on the forehead and readjusting the pillow more snugly around her shoulders. "Your offering is like gold, Mom—priceless. Nothing you are going through is a waste in God's eyes."

But even after her extraordinary grace, there were many days when Mom needed encouragement. The hours, days, and months spent immobile in her room, often seemed endless, and constituted the bulk of her bodily and spiritual sacrifice. At times it was intensely trying. Little by little, I learned more of the details.

"I especially miss reading," she told me one afternoon, reaching for the TV remote control on her bed table. "Reading was always my favorite thing in the world to do."

I crawled up behind her on the mattress, reached under her arms, and pulled her lighter-weight body higher up on the mattress.

"Thanks," she said. "Sometimes it feels like I'm lying in a hole down there."

"I remember the days when there were five or six books stacked on your bed table. Everything from politics to religion, science fiction to the writings of the mystics. You read them all."

"That's right," Mom said. "And I loved them. I read an entire book in a day if I could hide from you kids."

Chuckles.

I stepped off the bed and watched as she aimed the remote control. An old black-and-white movie flashed onto the TV screen.

Books are too heavy for her to hold open in bed now . . . I've tried everything . . . paperbacks, magazines, special shelves, raising the bed . . . she can't read in the wheelchair anymore; her eyes get too tired. Is there something else I haven't tried? No, I guess not . . .

Mom hit the mute button, her mind still on books. "I really loved the writings of the mystics. Have you ever read Julian of Norwich? It's up on the top bookshelf in Bill's room."

Watching TV or listening to tapes had become reading substitutes for Mom, providing interest and some entertainment. But there were many days when she was too tired even for that. Then she closed her eyes and lay motionless, given up to what seemed the sheer drudgery of nothingness.

"Are you okay?" I asked early one evening, noticing her TV off. I sensed a deeper, more somber quietude within her.

She didn't open her eyes. Answering in a faint monotone, she finally said, "I'm just tired. I feel so useless."

I knelt down and gently stroked her forehead. The feel of her silver strands were like silk under my fingertips. "You're not useless, Mom. Remember how you stroked my forehead this way when I was little? I always felt loved by you then, and still do. Your love does me a lot of good."

Whether my words helped to alleviate any of her bleak moments, I never knew. Still, I tried to ease some of her boredom by occasionally taking her out to do errands with me. In the late mornings, I often took her grocery shopping, and let her tote the plastic shopping basket in her lap. She enjoyed making purchasing suggestions, then handed each item to me at the checkout stand. She carried the filled shopping bag in her lap to the car, happy to feel "useful." Other times, I took her shopping for clothes. Whether the items were for her or for me, in a glance she sized up several garments, then pointed to the best one. "That." She was always right.

But it was the beach that lured Mom's spirit, the setting which most expanded her hemmed-in existence. I often took her to the waterfront in nearby Edmonds where I guided her along the paved walkway.

One day, gazing out over Puget Sound, her hair blowing slightly in the saltwater breeze, she described her growing years in upstate New York.

"I loved the rolling hills, and soft, sandy beaches," she said, referring to times that her father took the children on camping trips, or on short, daytime outings during the summer. "We waded out into the pretty lakes of the Adirondak Mountains and never felt a rock under our feet. We spent hours rowing around in little boats."

When she and Dad moved to the Northwest in 1948, they traveled by car, awestruck as they drove over Snoqualmie Pass and experienced the grandeur of the mountains for the first time.

"It was such a change to see rugged mountains and beaches," Mom said. "Everything was so much steeper and rockier. But I eventually learned to love the way it is here, too."

On warmer days, I wheeled her out onto a long dock in Edmonds and stopped at the far end. Beyond the protective rockery of a large marina, Mom looked west toward the Olympic Mountains, ignoring the local fisherman whose poles, buckets, and other fishing paraphernalia were strewn all around us. She either meditated silently, or spoke fondly of family trips over the same waters.

"Remember all of those ferry rides up to Ft. Flagler?" She looked to her right as one of the huge green-

and-white vessels suddenly blasted its horn, announcing departure from a nearby pier. All around, squawking seagulls swooped and soared into the cloudless sky, like pilots gliding upon avenues of wind.

"Those were great times," I said, visualizing the unforgettable family scenes.

Piled into an old, Chevy station wagon, we resembled something like a packed jelly bean jar, complete with stringed instruments and luggage. *Those were wonderful days. We were together as a family. It's been a long time.*

"Then there was you," I teasingly reminded Mom, watching as the sleek ferry pulled away from the dock, leaving a luscious white wake in its path. "You unfailingly hauled the Electrolux vacuum cleaner, mops, brooms, and Clorox along. I bet they took up half the car."

She chuckled, aware of her reputation for cleanliness, nothing to kid about in those days. No germ could withstand Mom's meticulous scrubbing. As soon as the car came to a halt in front of our primitive lodgings, Mom unpacked the cleaning gear and led the way to the first dirty floor.

"I'll never forget it," a female faculty member from the music festival remarked years later, reminiscing about Mom and her cleaning exuberance. "There was Agatha stepping from the car with vacuum cleaner, mops, and bleach in tow. You could smell it for days afterward."

But as much as Mom enjoyed these brief, afternoon interludes, she was happy to return home. As I helped her back into bed, she always said, "Thanks for taking me with you. I needed that." Closing her eyes, she said, "It's so nice to see something besides these four walls."

Alike to a monastic cell, Mom's room became her

sacred space with God. She made it so by the offering of her inner life, boredom and illness included. Every day she maintained a prayer regimen: one hour in the morning to pray the Rosary, two hours in the afternoon for listening to spiritual tapes, and two hours in the evening for prayer book devotions and private prayer. This followed upon no suggestion of mine. She was naturally drawn into the pattern.

"Quiet, please," she said, cutting off a question I began to ask while entering her room one evening.

For an hour, her light had been off, so I came to check on her.

"I'm not finished saying my prayers," she explained, glancing up. "Come back in about 15 minutes."

When I returned, I gently nudged. "May I ask how you were praying, Mom? At night, you always seem to have something very definite at heart."

"I do. I have about a hundred people I pray for by name every night before I go to sleep."

"A hundred?" Stunned, I listened as she continued.

"It makes me feel so good to know that I can do something for my friends."

"You are doing something, Mom. More than you know."

She smiled.

Her faith, fortified by grace, was unwavering. Yet, she harbored an overriding fear and occasionally shared it with me.

One evening, while lying in bed, she was peering through the bottom of her glasses, reading the 15 meditations of St. Bridget—"My fifteen," she called them—in a prayer booklet. For the same number of years, she had offered the inspired reflections each evening.

"What are they about?" I asked, one by one lifting items from her bed table away and setting them aside on the chest. I removed the towel covering, stained by apricot juice spilled earlier in the day, and replaced it with a fresh one. I adjusted the lamp and replaced the black portable radio.

Mom set her booklet aside, and answered, "They're meditations on the Passion of Christ in preparation for the moment of death. But, you know, I'm really afraid to face the moment of death."

"Why is that?" I stopped, turning to face her.

"Because I think I'll panic—just be completely terrified of what I have to face."

Her wide, childlike eyes reflected fierce honesty.

"Well, it has crossed my mind about how you might go, Mom." I took her hand. "And I don't think it will be anything horrible."

"Really?" She squeezed my hand.

"Of course. Someday, you'll just go poof."

Relaxing, she smiled at the quiet, high-pitched pronunciation of "poof."

I went on. "You're too tiny and cute for anything else. When the moment arrives, Jesus will come gently. You'll see."

Against the backdrop of the clamorous, often raging world, Mom's limited existence, lived out in the quiet seclusion of her room, provided a clarion perspective. Life was whittled down to the essentials, set squarely on the "straight and narrow" path to eternity.

Just exactly how do we measure love and the value of

relationships? What brings true happiness, self-knowledge, and peace?

As I reflected on these thoughts, St. Thérèse of Liseaux, the young, late 19th century Carmelite, was my caregiving inspiration, who described her experiences lucidly in her autobiography. One year, Thérèse was assigned to care for a cranky, elderly nun, and led the feeble woman to the refectory each evening. Responding with smiles rather than with retorts to the her unreasonable patient's demands, Thérèse soon discovered a great truth:

"One winter night I was carrying out my little duty as usual; it was cold, it was night. Suddenly, I heard off in the distance the harmonious sound of a musical instrument. I then pictured a well-lighted drawing room, brilliantly gilded, filled with elegantly dressed young ladies conversing together and conferring upon each other all sorts of compliments and other worldly remarks. Then my glance fell upon the poor invalid whom I was supporting. Instead of the beautiful strains of music I heard only her occasional complaints, and instead of the rich gildings I saw only the bricks of our austere cloister, hardly visible in the faintly glimmering light. I cannot express in words what happened in my soul; what I know is that the Lord illumined it with rays of *truth* which so surpassed the dark brilliance of earthly feasts that I could not believe my happiness." (from *Story of a Soul,* St. Thérèse of Lisieux)

Like Thérèse, I also experienced a similar joy while caring for Mom. Though able to go out and play occasional music jobs, which became possible again after two years, I always looked forward to returning home again.

The pure love of our relationship was like a star in the night, providing healing and strength.

One night, upon returning home from a particularly substandard gig, I walked through the back door and heard Mom's familiar greeting. "Hi!"

"Hi, Tiny," I responded, continuing the ritual as I set down my violin case and walked down the hallway.

Her gentle ambiance greeted me as I entered the room, offset by the white glow of the bedspread in the darkness. Quietly, she asked, "How did it go?"

"Not well," I sighed, hating to ruin the peaceful atmosphere. "Bad music. Bad conductor. It's hard to take."

"Here, lie down," she said, patting the right side of the bedspread.

Sinking down next to her, I slipped my hand into hers.

"Just offer it up, Little One. Everything will be fine."

"Do you really think so?" Silently I prayed, releasing my burden.

Turning slightly, Mom looked toward her trees, her inward gaze upon God.

Preparations and Song

By the beginning of 1997, Mom's condition had changed. Over the course of the previous year, due to a diminished appetite, her weight had dropped significantly, creating a daily challenge to get enough food and liquid into her.

"Drink, Mom," I said, seated next to her at the kitchen table one afternoon, holding a small, brown-tinted glass to her lips. Already, I had waited the better part of 30 minutes as she nibbled half of a BLT sandwich. I anticipated the same amount of time for her to drink a mere four ounces of water. Without my continual goading, the water would simply be left.

"I'm not thirsty," she said, though obediently upending the glass and swallowing the last few tablespoons just to please me. She handed it back. "Now may I get down?" She closed her eyes, overcome with weariness.

Decreased energy meant less activity for Mom. No more did she spend a pleasant hour after meals watching TV in the kitchen. No longer did she attend Mass on Sunday, or accompany me on several outings during the week. When Dad treated us to dinner at a restaurant, which was almost every Sunday evening, Mom couldn't relax at the table. She complained of a sore back, squirming with pain, and plied the armrest, uninterested in conversation.

"We need to go home," I would finally inform Dad,

motioning for a waiter to come. We made our retreat hastily, carrying Mom's barely picked-at food in a box.

Later, in the spring of that same year, Mom was beset with a new challenge, though of a much heavier sort. She contracted a mysterious stomach ailment, which none of the doctors could diagnose. She suffered from constant nausea, telling me, "I feel like I'm pregnant again," and never felt like eating. The little nourishment I did coax into her never sat well, and I found myself more and more spoon-feeding her like an infant.

"Here, let me do that, Mom."

Seated at dinner one evening, she misjudged the distance to her mouth, and the soup dribbled from the spoon, running down her chin onto the napkin. Lowering the spoon back into the bowl, she looked up with childlike innocence. "I guess I missed. Could you help?"

Taking over, I fed her the rest of the soup, then quietly left the room. Months of witnessing her gradual diminishment had caught up with me, and I poured out my heart in tears. *She's getting more and more helpless. How far will it go? It's so hard to see her this way . . .*

The ponderous atmosphere increased as I left Mom's room a few weeks later and found Dad sitting near the dining room window, reading a book.

Not his usual reading place, or time.

Knowing he had probably delved into the book's far-removed contents as a way to cope with his emotional burden, I said, "Dad?" hoping conversation might offer some relief. Intensely withdrawn, however, he didn't look up.

Leave him be.

At the moment, there seemed to be no escape from our trial.

A phone call later that same afternoon brought an unexpected ray of sunshine. Picking up the receiver, I held the phone to my ear and heard the caller say, "Hi, Jenny!"

Stunned, I recognized the voice, but wondered, *Can it be?* Sure enough, from the cloister, my sister Claire, a Carmelite nun, was phoning from the monastery for the first time in years. In those days, family phone calls and home visits were rare in Carmel.

"Why are you calling?" I asked, thrilled to communicate with her in a normal way. "It's so good to hear your voice. But is something wrong?"

"Oh, no," Claire answered, beginning to chuckle. "It's just that I really need to talk to Dad. Is he home?"

"No, not right now. Can I give him a message?"

"Sure," she replied, "But let me tell you what's happened. I've volunteered to write a song for the Carmelite Order in honor of St. Thérèse's centenary of death. You know, the celebration that's coming up this September?"

"Yes."

"Well, at first I thought I would only write a one-line melody with keyboard accompaniment. Really simple, right? But now I'm hearing something much bigger."

"Like what?"

She began to laugh as the rest of her idea spilled out. "I'm going to write a song for a large mixed choir, plus instrumentation! Can you believe this? It means I have to write a score, but I don't know how to. I really need Dad's help. Could you please ask him to call?"

I smiled, confident of Claire's talent. "Of course. But I have to tell you that all of this is happening at the right moment. Mom is going through a really difficult time, and this is just the boost we need. When Dad gets home, I'll give him the message. Everything will work out, I'm sure."

The next few weeks turned into a whirlwind, musical collaboration between Claire and Dad. Under pressure to meet a recording deadline, she spent all of her spare time composing. Each day she left pages of manuscript at the front door of the monastery and Dad picked them up to study at home.

Often, emerging from his room in the morning, he stood in the doorway, and announced, "I thought of a wonderful new chord last night! I'll have to let Claire know about it right away." Energized, he made his way to the piano in the living room where he played his overnight discoveries. Afterward, he phoned Claire. "Wolfgang?" They laughed, amused by the nickname he had chosen, an allusion to the great Mozart. Humor filled every conversation.

Mom's spirits also lifted. "This is just what your father needs," she said, hearing the back door close one afternoon as Dad headed over to the monastery. Her eyes, usually clouded over from nausea, were lit with a healthier glow. "He needs something creative."

I sat down on the bed and picked up her cup, filled with fresh apricot juice. "Please, take another sip, Mom."

She smiled, still thinking of Dad. "It's nice he has something to think about besides me."

But I grew more curious about Mom. With so much talk about a song these days, I wondered about her own vocal background, that mostly unknown area of her life, which had always seemed like her "first love" in music to me. Before marrying, she was an accomplished violinist and performed in various orchestras. But she also sang in fine choirs and taught singing to children in elementary public schools. Dad had gained an international reputation as a conductor. But what about Mom? Had she also known days on the podium? Perhaps she was comfortable enough to share her story with me.

My opportunity arose as I carried a stack of folded laundry into her room one morning.

Seeing me pass by, she pulled away the headphone from her ear and commented about the choral CD she was listening to. "It's so delicate. You should hear this, Jenny. I wish I could sing like that again."

"You will in heaven, Mom." The sound of her light soprano voice floated through my memory. I pulled open the top dresser drawer. "In heaven, your beautiful voice will return, better than ever."

One by one, I set the clean garments inside the drawer. Without turning, I asked, "I know you taught singing to children after college. But what about adults? Did you ever conduct an adult choir?"

To my surprise, Mom set aside all previous reticence, laughing heartily as she said, "Yes, and your father was in one of them in the Army."

"The Army?" I spun around, enthralled. "You conducted Dad in the Army?"

Delighted, Mom described the small military choir, which she formed at the request of a Protestant chaplain in Biloxi. "Nothing great," she admitted. "But it was enough to accompany the Sunday service; that's all he wanted. Since your father had a musical background, I begged him to join the group. I just needed sound."

"Did you conduct other choirs before the Army, then? Good ones, I mean?"

"Yes," Mom answered, lowering her voice, aware of her private past. "At one time, I was considered the music leader in upstate New York."

"Really?" I backed up, slowly pushing the dresser drawer closed behind me. Holding her gaze, I folded my arms and considered the depth of her musical prowess, more significant than I had ever realized. "So why did you stop conducting? You could have formed a group in Seattle. Were you trying to be the humble wife or something?"

"I just knew that your father was a great man, and was meant to be in the spotlight, so I gave it up."

Her manner, as unobtrusive as her long-ago resolution, was devoid of regret. From the day she resolved to lay down the baton, she never wavered. Her whole life became a gift for Dad and the family.

But the "choral conductor" in her remained, and I caught a glimpse of it a few mornings later. That was the day Claire came home to play her nearly completed composition for us, entitled *Thérèse's Canticle of Love*. Claire was especially thinking about Mom, who would not be able to attend the recording session of the Cathedral Choir at St. James Cathedral in May. As an added blessing, Mom's stomach ailment disappeared that morning. Though weak, she sat up, ate a normal breakfast, then waited for Claire.

A quiet knock sounded at the back door.

"Hi!" Claire said, greeting Dad and me in the doorway. She strode around the corner into the kitchen, setting her brown canvas bag down on the floor. As she warmly embraced Mom, fifteen years of her absence came together in an instant—having her home seemed perfectly natural.

"It's wonderful to see you, Claire," Mom said, looking up. "Thank you for coming."

Camera in hand, Dad was already snapping photos. "Now, let's get one of the three of you together." He directed Claire and me into exact positions beside Mom. "How about a smile from all of you lovely girls?" He adjusted the lens.

"But we can't leave Mom sitting up too long," I cautioned, whispering into Claire's ear. "She just started feeling better this morning. I don't want to push it."

"Got it." Photo session complete, Claire lifted three sheets of song text from her bag. Handing them to us, she walked down into the living room and she sat down at the piano. She was visible to all of us from the kitchen. Dad stood near Mom at the table, and I walked to the sink to fill a glass of water. Turning, I remained there, curious to view Mom's response from a distance. *What will it be?*

The piano introduction began. Phrase by phrase, Claire's melody filled the house, touching our hearts with beauty and with God's love. "Oh, come to the living water," a verse read, "fear not your weakness, forever trusting in God's merciful love . . ."

Reaching the end, Claire stopped and waited for comments. "What do you think?"

Dad was first. "It's beautiful, honey. Really beautiful. I love the way the harmonies move from one to the next. But the ending really needs to be held back. Do you know what I'm talking about?" He demonstrated, humming the phrase as he conduced the ritard with strong gestures.

Mimicking on the piano, Claire agreed and reached for her pencil to mark in the change. "And what about you, Mom? Do you have anything to say?"

Slowly, Mom extended her right arm out in front of her, angling the hand and fingers just so, ready to give the downbeat.

The choral conductor! I held my breath.

"You know those eighth notes in the piano part at the very beginning," she said, her voice soft but confident. "And how they return at the end?"

She remembered every note.

"Yes," Claire replied.

"I hear 'Alleluias' there." Gently, she conducted the phrase, speaking each word. As if they were always meant to be, she slowly lowered her arm.

"Mmm . . . lovely," Claire said, absorbing the inspired idea. She lifted her pencil and inscribed the new text into the score. "Thanks, Mom. That's perfect."

Two weeks later, Claire stood in the west end of the cathedral, anxiously waiting for the evening recording session to begin. Would the voicing be correct? The instrumentation complimentary to the choir? Would the harp be audible? And the strings as well? All of these concerns tumbled through her mind as she prepared to hear the debut of her composition.

"I couldn't believe my ears," she told me later, "when the choir came in. Their incredible sound within those acoustics was even more beautiful than I had imagined."

To complete her dream, Dad stood on the podium that night, holding the baton. Dr. James Savage, the cathedral's music director and former conducting student of my father, had graciously extended the conducting invitation to his teacher.

"Dad brought out things in the music I never realized were there before," Claire said. "It was like hearing my piece on another level."

Earlier, in the fall of the previous year, Dad had joined the cathedral as a parishioner. With the emergence of *Thérèse's Canticle of Love*, the cathedral's liturgical life and music became an integral part of our journey at home. Dad shared inspiring stories about the liturgy each week, and Mom listened daily to her *Canticle* tape.

"Only for today," she said, rearticulating Thérèse's words, which recurred as a prayerful motif throughout the song.

Standing at the foot of Mom's bed, I reached under the covers and tugged at the bottom of her pant legs. As usual, the knit fabric had bunched up beneath her knees.

"Thanks," she said, adjusting the volume on the tape machine and returning to her musical prayer. Absorbed in the melody, she repeated the same words like a mantra: "Only for today."

Yes, only for the next five minutes.

Two months later, on the first day of July, I stood on the steps of St. James. The hot sun filtered through a thin cloud cover, and I gazed at a brown casket set on the cement landing several feet below. Surrounded by Native Americans dressed in traditional costumes, and holding folk-like drums, the austere wooden container was a sharp contrast to their colorful panache. With the rest of us, the native musicians were there to participate in The Rite of Reception into the cathedral of Archbishop Thomas J. Murphy, who died at the end of June.

My thoughts traveled back, recalling the unexpected letter, which he sent to me several months after I left Carmel. The personal gesture was a beacon of comfort during that difficult time. Now I prayed, *Please help me when the time comes to say good-bye to Mom. But most of all, help her, however she needs it.*

Just then, I looked up and recognized a man standing just ahead of me, a priest. Seeing his head bowed, and hands crossed in front of him, I suspected he too was praying. Gently, I touched his shoulder. *Will he recognize me? The last time he saw me was in Carmel.*

He turned.

"Hi, Monsignor Doogan." Recognizing the blank stare which followed, I clarified my identity. "I'm Jenny Sokol."

"Oh, yes, Jenny." He took my hand. "How are you?

I explained about Mom and our situation at home. Then he began to share anecdotes of standing on these same steps many times before. He gestured with his hand between the casket and the cathedral building, describing the installations and funerals of former prelates, some from as far back as his childhood. He described his own ordination at St. James and the many changes that had taken place since then. To him, every inch of the limestone brick structure held a rich story, etched in history.

Fascinated by his knowledge and at ease in his company, I knew Mom would feel the same way. *Perhaps he would agree to visit her.*

"Monsi—"

But he didn't hear me. The low-pitched drums began to beat, breaking the silence. All eyes turned, riveted on the casket.

Then, as the Native Americans began to chant their special invocations, Monsignor turned with the crowd and began to process into the cathedral.

I guess I can find someone else—

Suddenly, he turned and faced me again. "Jenny, if there's anything I can ever do for you, please let me know."

I had my chance. "There is one thing."

"Yes?"

"For weeks, Mom has been asking for a priest to hear her confession. Do you think you could come to our home? She's not able to get out to church anymore."

"Of course," he replied. "Anytime."

During the next year, Monsignor Doogan visited Mom four times. After each visit she always summarized her experience in exactly the same words, "He gives me so much peace."

Gradually, I recognized that a spiritual preparation was underway. While Mom spent more time in prayer, preparing to meet her Maker, I accepted more violin work in preparation to let her go. But if two jobs fell on the same day, I only agreed to play both if I could return home in between and check on Mom. Seeing me, we chatted as I adjusted her covers, helped her onto the commode, or sat next to her on the bed. My mere presence was enough to say, "I'm still here," and she never worried, feeling safe.

I made other small preparations as well, pulling up stakes from my living room "camp" and moving back into my room. There were more serious episodes as well, which prepared me for her death.

One afternoon, as I stood next to her in the kitchen after lunch, I was trying to decide whether or not to take a walk. I wondered, *Will she be safe without me? Or should I wait until Dad gets home?*

But Mom urged me to go. "You need to get some fresh air." She pointed toward the window. "See, it's not raining anymore, and the walk will do you good."

"All right," I said, putting on my jacket and walking toward the back door. "I'll just pick up the order at the pharmacy and be back in 25 minutes, no more."

Once down the hill, though, second thoughts crept in. *Maybe Mom is tiring. She might be panicked . . . or desperate to lie down. Maybe I shouldn't have left! Oh, God . . .*

Carrying the prescriptions, I rushed from the pharmacy and headed for the pay phone in the parking lot. I dialed home, agonizing as I listened to several unanswered rings go by. *Won't they stop? Endless! Why doesn't Mom answer?*

Ring, ring . . .

Oh, God, is she dead? It's my fault!

I shoved the phone back down and alternated between walking and running as I hiked back up the steep hill. My heart pounded like a bass drum. Reaching the top, I ran down the driveway and charged through the back door. I called out, "Mom?" terrified that I wouldn't hear an answer.

Then it came. "Yes?" Seated around the corner, she was just where I had left her, waiting calmly as if nothing had happened.

Panting, I dropped my jacket to the floor, already shed halfway up the hill, and ran to her side. "Why didn't you pick up the phone? I tried to call you, but you didn't answer. I thought you were dead!"

"I did hear it ring," she said. "But it was on the table

next to the back door. I couldn't steer fast enough around the corner to get it."

I started to cry, releasing both trauma and relief at the same time.

"There," Mom said, pointing to one of the kitchen table chairs. "Why don't you pull it over and put your head down." She patted her wheelchair tray.

I dragged the chair over and sat down, laying my cheek on the tray. "I'm sorry, Mom. I guess I didn't give you the phone before I left. I thought I did."

"Don't worry, nothing happened. But remember, if you ever do come home and find me dead, just thank God."

"Thank God?" I sat up, amazed by her faith. "Do you really think it will be that easy for me?"

Laying my head back down, I looked out the window. The rain was falling again and gently pattered against the roof. Soothed by the sound, I closed my eyes and visualized a scene, one that I had pictured a thousand times before:

It was night, and I walked into Mom's room where I found her dead. Unemotional, I gazed at her lifeless figure in the darkened room and knew her soul had been taken during sleep. I then walked into Dad's room, determined not to cry, and informed him of the horrid news.

I'll thank God, just like Mom said. Yes, I'll be strong, courageous, and handle everything like a pillar of practicality. A saint!

But deeper, I couldn't deny my heart. How could I possibly hope to protect myself from love and its fathomless cost at that moment? I couldn't even do that during our normal routine together. Each day, I loved Mom even more, tangibly felt as I walked into her room and caught sight of her sweet face. My heart swelled. "It feels like a balloon!" I often told her, holding my hands over my heart. "This is how much I love you, Mom. You're just so tiny and cute!"

Sitting up in the kitchen now, I faced her, ready to face reality. "I can't promise perfect composure when you die. But if you pray for me, no matter what, I'll have the grace I need. Will you do that?"

"Yes, of course. Every day I pray that nice things will come into your life."

Soon afterward, in the fall of 1997, I joined The Women of St. James Schola, a small chant choir at the cathedral. Each Sunday evening I returned home following the Schola's 5:30 Mass and shared the musical highlights with Mom.

"You're lucky to be in a group like that," she said, looking up from her pillow on an evening in December, the feast of Our Lady of Guadalupe. "Mary is taking care of you."

"Yes," I agreed, reaching under Mom's shoulders and lifting her. Prepared for the Sunday evening shower, I helped her onto the commode, put her shower gown on, and wheeled her across the hallway into the bathroom.

I continued to describe the music. "At the Offertory, we sang a beautiful two-part setting of a psalm, nothing I've ever heard before." I positioned the commode in front of the sink and bent, setting the brakes. "You would have loved it, Mom." I straightened, picked up the toothbrush, squeezed on some toothpaste, and handed it to her. "Maybe you could come and hear us sing sometime. Would you like that?"

I looked at her through her reflection in the mirror and watched as she opened her mouth to reply. Suddenly, her speech became indistinct—*Garbled!*—and her words wouldn't form. Recognizing the unmistakable symptom of a stroke, I froze, wondering, *Will it pass?*

Terrified, Mom stared back, helplessly groping the sink ledge as she struggled to speak. But the words remained muddled.

"Don't try to talk anymore," I finally said, reaching around and gently covering her mouth with my right hand. "Just relax."

I leaned down and embraced her, at the same moment hearing a quiet thought: *Invite the Schola to come to the house* .

Yes, Mom may not make it to next Christmas.

Still holding her, I suggested, "Why don't we just silently say a Hail Mary together, Mom. I think it will help."

Finished with my prayer, I stood. "Do you feel strong enough to take a shower?

She nodded.

"All right, then. Let's keep doing the same thing, and not talk."

The next half hour was spent in complete silence. Mom completed the transfer into the shower, and moved about as usual. Back in her room, she dried her hair with the hair dryer, then laid it back down on the mattress.

I stepped in front of her, and asked, "Can you talk now?"

"Yes."

"Thank God." Relieved to hear distinct words, I leaned down and hugged her. "Let's do the transfer now."

The Schola came to sing for Mom the day after Christmas. With members of our family, the occasion was a holiday gathering. My sisters and I played string quartets before dinner, then afterward the Schola gathered around Mom's bed to sing. Among others works, we sang Praetorius's joyful *Regina Coeli*. The sound of high treble voices filled the room, and my little nieces and nephews stood, mesmerized, listening in the doorway. Surrounded by adults, they had never seen or heard such an event in our home. None of us would ever forget this incredibly beautiful concert.

Especially Mom. Later, when everyone had left, she told me, "High treble voices are the song of my heart." Her face, glowing radiantly, seemed to light the darkness.

Noticing this phenomena more and more, I wondered, *How much closer can she come to God before departing this earth? Will she divulge her interior secret?*

Finally, one night, I asked, "What are you smiling about, Mom?"

Shyly she looked away, like a young girl in love. Then, beginning to laugh softly, she looked toward the ceiling, her eyes bright with joy. "Oh, nothing, really."

"Nothing?"

But I knew—God.

Memories in the Waves

I am at the Edmonds waterfront and step down from the walkway onto the beach. The mid-afternoon sun in May plays on the wet sand, feigning a burnished cobalt carpet for my feet. Walking in white sneakers, I take in the brisk saltwater air and enjoy the pleasant breeze, which brushes my face. Seaweed clumps, lying in shallow pools, are scattered every several yards, and rocks, embedded beneath my feet, are flattened like tiny saucers. Aligned with the sand's surface, their smoothness reflects the age-less flow of waves over them.

I look up now and smile at a fat seagull, which stands and stares back at me from its pebbly post by the water's edge. *This is why I love it here, and why Mom loved it, too.* I savor the raw, unpretentious beauty, which surrounds my web-footed friend, and listen to the sound of the waves as they crest, gently releasing their watery burden at the shore.

I hear Mom's voice again, soft and clear: "I hope I can enjoy my heaven without you."

Spoken a few months before her death, six years ago, they are chiseled in my heart, offering quiet assurance of her presence. Her words imply that she is thinking of me, and that even in her blissful state, somehow she misses me, too. We are still together.

Another wave reaches its destination and tumbles

freely, washing ashore. Just so, another memory wells up within, rising like the seagull, which suddenly launches from the sea foam and raises a piercing cry toward heaven: "Please pray that Jesus will come," Mom had said.

Startled by the directness of her request, I inquired, "Are you asking that for me or for you?"

"For you," she responded weakly, fingering her beads as she lay in bed that evening in Lent. Without opening her eyes, she clarified her meaning. "I'm in your way."

"You're not in my way, Mom. Please, don't think that."

But she was certain. "Just pray."

Suddenly, I felt pushed to the limit. Words of prayer caught in my throat and my heart jammed shut, resisting what I feared would surely be answered if I did pray.

Confused and frustrated, I left Mom's room and walked down to mine. Sitting on the edge of my bed, I sifted through my thoughts, overwhelmed. I tried to rationalize, determined to avoid granting Mom's request. *After all, praying for her death would be selfish and cruel . . . isn't that right, Jesus? I love her and want her to live. Isn't it wrong for me to pray for her death? Of course it is . . . that's what you think . . . I know it is . . . at least, I think I do . . .*

But deeper, I knew that I didn't want to let Mom go—ever. And that, it began to dawn on me, was my greatest conflict. So I prayed to be able to pray—according to Mom's request—with my eyes closed, head bowed, arms folded, silently agonizing as I rocked there for one hour on the edge of my bed.

When the storm finally passed, my mind quieted and peace settled within. I opened my eyes and gave my consent. "Jesus, please come and take Mom to heaven. That's what she wants, and I give her to you."

A week has now passed since my last visit to the waterfront and the waves beckon as I step from my car and approach the beach. Drawing nearer, I zip my jacket higher, then suddenly halt as I catch sight of the beach. Puzzled, I stare at a thick, mottled layer of seaweed strewn across the full length of the sandy expanse. I wonder, *How could last week's silvery sheen now be transformed into a picture of chaos?* Then I remember: *The storm.*

An unexpected tempest had raged through the area a few days previously, downing trees and knocking out power lines. Witnessing the aftermath, I understand that a natural purgation has taken place. The waves have merely cooperated in their part of the process and revealed the sea's hidden depths.

Like the morning I found Mom . . . a shocking revelation.

Contrary to the composed manner I had imagined for myself in my recurring daydream, I peeked through her doorway that morning and gasped, horrified. I stared at her ashen figure, unable to believe what I was seeing, and called out, "Mom? Mom?" hoping to hear an answer. When it never came, I began to tremble. I walked to her motionless side and peered at her face, her pale lips offset by a trickle of dried blood following down the right corner. I wondered, *Can it be?* Dreading what I must do next, I reached down and took her pallid cheeks in my hands. *Ice cold!* It was true. Stepping back, I stared into the ghastly hue covering the once-beautiful countenance of my mother, and began to wail.

"*. . . the waves of death swept round me.*" (2 Samuel 22:5, NEB)

The words of scripture return as I gaze across the wind-whipped waves, accented by leaping white caps.

The waves of Mom's death swept round me . . . like a flood . . . but there were clear signs beforehand.

"I had a dream last night," she told me, two mornings before she died.

"Oh, really?" Curious to hear the details, I stood by her bed holding the water basin, prepared to wash her. I set the basin on the floor and rolled her onto her side, laying the bath towel underneath. I asked, "Was it another funny one? I can hardly wait to hear."

"No," Mom replied, humorless. "I dreamt I was in a room filled with coffins."

I stiffened at the morose implication and met her serious gaze. "That's not so nice."

No comment.

The dream's sober imagery stayed with me the rest of the morning. What did it mean? Was Mom depressed? Thinking of someone else's death? Or perhaps her own? She didn't expound any further, so neither did I. I set aside all questions and carried on with my chores as usual, hoping the subject would simply fade away and be forgotten, like a fleeting rain drizzle or a tiny wave.

But death was right at the door . . . Mom's spirit already knew that, and so did her body.

The evening following her dream, she faltered in the shower and nearly doubled over on the shower bench. I struggled to pull her upright, but felt her lack of strength.

"Please, Mom, I won't be able to transfer you out

of the shower if you can't hold yourself up. Can you help me?"

"I'm trying," she said, lifting her head as she struggled to reach the arm rail. "I feel so weak. I don't know why."

Confused by the sudden, inexplicable decline in her condition, I prayed, poised on the edge of panic. *Jesus, I won't be able to take care for her at home if she gets much weaker.*

Gratefully, she was able to transfer out of the shower and revived by the time she was back in bed. Her eyes were bright and her face radiated joy. Sitting down on the chest, I lifted a skirt, which was laid over the dresser, and methodically began to stitch the hem into place.

Dad and my sister Paula, who was visiting from Michigan, joined us in the room and began to chat. We shared many family memories and often laughed hysterically. Still, I was preoccupied. *What's wrong with Mom? The dream . . . coffins . . . so weak in the shower . . . something is out of kilter.*

Later, before leaving her for the final time that evening, I began to cough from a bad cold, so Mom offered the same advice she had always given to me when I was young.

"Please, put the vaporizer by your bed."

"No, thanks." I coughed into my arm again. "I'll be fine. I just need to rest."

Her smile glowed as she reached up and pulled me down to herself. "I love you so much. Thank you for everything."

"You're welcome, Mom."

That was the last thing I saw . . . her radiant smile . . . then death . . .

Standing next to her motionless figure the next morning, I wiped my tears, frantically looking around in search of a clue—anything that would indicate the cause of her death. *Did she have a stroke? Or choke during a coughing spell?* But all I noticed were her undisturbed blankets and everything on the bed table arranged neatly in order, just as she had left them the night before.

Like her soul—perfectly in order, ready to meet God.

Her right hand rested on her tummy, unmoved during the night. Her rosary was draped softly between her fingers.

She was not alone. Mary was with her . . .

Still trembling, I walked into Dad's room, my thoughts shrouded by death, and told him about Mom.

"Oh, my God," he said. "I'll be right there."

Walking into Paula's room downstairs, I stood, dazed and crying at the foot of her bed. Hearing my shocking news, she bolted upright and nearly flew from beneath her covers. A minute later we were standing with Dad alongside Mom.

How I wished her eyelids would open, defying death . . .

Suddenly, Paula laid her right hand on my shoulder, and said, "Jenny, Mom is in heaven!"

The Resurrection! I had forgotten.

Paula's reminder was like a light breaking through the gloom, much like the sunshine, which now breaks through the clouds and dapples the turbulent water. Sweeping across the beach, it lights the confusion and takes the edge off the day's windy chill. At that moment, I think of the angel who enlightened the bewildered women at Jesus' empty tomb: "Remember what he said to you . . . that the Son of Man must be . . . crucified, and on the third day rise again." (Luke 24:6–7, NAB)

Paula was like an angel who gave me hope. But there was another angel . . . at Mom's funeral.

The liturgy, attended by several hundred people, took place on a sunlit morning at St. James Cathedral. I sat with the family near Mom's casket and remembered her once lonely existence. Could she have imagined the number of people who would gather that day, or the musical beauty that would accompany her farewell liturgy, graced by a harp, a string quartet, a women's choir, and a pipe organ? I took in the sight of so many friends, and the inspired words of our pastor, Father Michael G. Ryan. At the end of the liturgy, the haunting chords of Duruflé's *In Paradisum* filled the cathedral, and the family slowly followed Mom's casket out through the north doors of the cathedral.

Tearful, a single memory lingered. *"Mom is a lamb."*

The thought had occurred to me about a year before her death. As I was helping her onto the commode, then back into bed one afternoon, I was saddened by her listless energy, which had persisted for weeks. Eyes closed, she whispered, "Thank you," and sank back onto the pillow. Reminded of the silent Lamb of God who lovingly laid down his life for his friends, I knew Mom was the living reflection.

I followed her casket now, as it turned onto the sidewalk of the cathedral, but I didn't notice the person standing nearby, who suddenly reached out and placed a greeting card in my hand. Misty-eyed, I stared at the name written on the envelope, then blinked. Had I read it correctly? It was addressed to Mom, but rather than her own name, Agatha, "Agnus" was inscribed instead, the Latin word for "lamb." Realizing God's merciful acknowledgement of my mother's total offering, I looked up to thank my unknown messenger—the "angel"—but no one was there.

At least, that I could see . . .

I turn away from the beach now, ready to return home. Beginning to walk, I hear the rushing of waves as a final memory returns, this time, my favorite.

"When I get to heaven," Mom had said, "I'm going to sit right next to Mary and talk about you all day."

"All day?" I asked, laughing.

Quickening my pace, I listen as the sound of waves fades into the distance.

Then that's where I'll stay, too, Mom—right next to Mary, where you are.